STUDENT LABORATORY MANUAL FOR

PHYSICAL
EXAMINATION
& HEALTH
ASSESSMENT

FOURTH EDITION

STUDENT LABORATORY MANUAL FOR

PHYSICAL
EXAMINATION
& HEALTH
ASSESSMENT

F O U R T H   E D I T I O N

CAROLYN JARVIS, MSN, APN, CNP

Family Nurse Practitioner
Chestnut Health Systems
Bloomington, Illinois
and
Adjunct Assistant Professor of Nursing
Illinois Wesleyan University
Bloomington, Illinois

SAUNDERS
An Imprint of Elsevier

An Imprint of Elsevier

11830 Westline Industrial Drive
St. Louis, Missouri 63146

Student Laboratory Manual for
PHYSICAL EXAMINATION AND HEALTH ASSESSMENT,
Fourth Edition
Copyright © 2004, 2000, 1996, Elsevier All Rights Reserved.

Notice

Nursing is an ever-changing field. Standard safety precautions must be followed, but as new research and clinical experience broaden our knowledge, changes in treatment and drug therapy may become necessary or appropriate. Readers are advised to check the most current product information provided by the manufacturer of each drug to be administered to verify the recommended dose, the method and duration of administration, and contraindications. It is the responsibility of the licensed health care provider, relying on experience and knowledge of the patient, to determine dosages and the best treatment for each individual patient. Neither the publisher nor the author assumes any liability for any injury and/or damage to persons or property arising from this publication.

THE PUBLISHER

International Standard Book Number 0-7216-9775-5

Executive Vice President, Nursing Health Professions: Sally Schrefer
Executive Publisher: Robin Carter
Developmental Editors: Deanna Davis, Kristin Geen
Editorial Assistant: Jamie Randall
Publishing Services Manager: Gayle May
Project Manager: Stephanie M. Hebenstreit
Senior Designer: Kathi Gosche

Printed in the United States of America.

Last digit is the print number: 9 8 7 6 5 4 3

Contributors

Jacquelyn C. Campbell, PhD, RN, FAAN
Anna D. Wolf Endowed Professor and Associate Dean for Faculty Affairs
School of Nursing
Johns Hopkins University
Baltimore, Maryland
* Co-contributor for Chapter 5: Domestic Violence Assessment

Jeannine Forrest, PhD, RN
Research Assistant Professor
Department of Medical and Surgical Nursing
University of Illinois
Chicago, Illinois
* Contributor for Chapter 11: Pain Assessment: The Fifth Vital Sign

Joyce K. Keithley, DNSc, RN, FAAN
Practitioner-Teacher and Professor
Rush-Presbyterian–St. Luke's Medical Center
Rush University College of Nursing
Chicago, Illinois
* Contributor for Chapter 8: Nutritional Assessment

Daniel J. Sheridan, PhD, RN, CNS
Assistant Professor and Forensic Clinical Nurse Specialist
School of Nursing
Johns Hopkins University
Baltimore, Maryland
* Co-contributor for Chapter 5: Domestic Violence Assessment

Deborah E. Swenson, BSN, ARNP
Perinatal Nurse Practitioner
OBSTETRIX Medical Group of Washington
Seattle, Washington
* Contributor for Chapter 27: The Pregnant Female

Preface

This Student Laboratory Manual is intended for you, the student, as a study guide and laboratory manual to accompany the textbook *Physical Examination and Health Assessment,* 4th edition. You will use it in two places: in your own study area and in the skills laboratory.

As a study guide, this workbook highlights and reinforces the content from the text. Each chapter corresponds to a chapter in the textbook and contains workbook exercises and questions in varying formats that provide the repetition needed to synthesize and master content from the text. Fill out the lab manual chapter and answer the questions before coming to the skills laboratory. This will reinforce your lectures, expose any areas needing questioning for your clinical instructor, and prime you for the skills laboratory/clinical experience.

Once in the skills laboratory, use the Student Laboratory Manual as a direct clinical tool. Each chapter contains assessment forms on perforated tear-out pages. Usually you will work in pairs and perform the regional physical examinations on each other under the tutelage of your instructor. As you perform the examination on your peer, you can fill out the write-up sheet and assessment form to be handed in and checked by the instructor.

Three new chapters have been added to the laboratory manual to accompany new material in the 4th edition textbook: Domestic Violence Assessment, Pain Assessment: The Fifth Vital Sign, and The Pregnant Female.

Features

Each chapter is divided into two parts, cognitive and clinical, and contains:

- Purpose—a brief summary of the material you are learning in this chapter
- Reading Assignment—the corresponding chapter and page numbers from the *Physical Examination and Health Assessment* textbook, and space for your instructor to assign journal articles
- Audio-Visual Assignment—the corresponding video assignment from the Saunders Video Physical Examination and Health Assessment Series, which is adapted from the *Physical Examination and Health Assessment* textbook, as well as space for your instructor to assign relevant audio tapes or computer-assisted learning modules
- Glossary—important and specialized terms from the textbook chapter with accompanying definitions
- Study Guide—specific short-answer and fill-in questions to help you highlight and learn content from the chapter. The critical thinking questions from the video assessment series are included to coordinate the reading and video assignments. Important art figures of human anatomy have been reproduced

from the textbook with the labels deleted so that you can identify and fill in the names of the structures yourself.

- Review Questions—new and revised multiple-choice questions, matching, and short-answer questions in a format similar to usual college classroom exams, so that you can monitor your own mastery of the material. Take the self-exam when you are ready and then check your answers against the correct answers given in Appendix A.
- Clinical Objectives—behavioral objectives that you should achieve during your peer practice in the regional examinations
- Regional Write-up Sheets—complete yet succinct physical examination forms that you can use in the skills lab or in the clinical setting. These serve as a memory prompt, listing key history questions and physical exam steps, and they serve as a means of recording data during the client encounter.
- Narrative Summary Forms—S O A P format, so that you can learn to chart narrative accounts of the history and physical exam findings. These forms have accompanying sketches of regional anatomy and are an especially useful exercise for those studying for advanced practice roles.

Learning the skills of history taking and physical examination requires two kinds of practice: cognitive and clinical. It is my hope that this Student Laboratory Manual will help you achieve both of these learning and practice modalities.

CAROLYN JARVIS

Acknowledgment

I am grateful to all those on the team at W.B. Saunders Company (Elsevier) who worked on the Student Laboratory Manual. My thanks extend to Robin Carter, Executive Publisher, Nursing, for her leadership, encouragement, and organizational support; and to Deanna Davis, Developmental Editor, and Stephanie Hebenstreit, Project Manager for their extreme helpfulness and for their guidance and coordination in various stages of production.

CAROLYN JARVIS

Contents

UNIT 1   Assessment of the Whole Person

UNIT 2   Approach to the Clinical Setting

UNIT 3   Physical Examination

UNIT 4   Integration of the Health Assessment

Appendixes

UNIT 1

Assessment of the Whole Person

CHAPTER 1

Critical Thinking in Health Assessment

PURPOSE

This chapter discusses the characteristics of diagnostic reasoning, the nursing process, and critical thinking. This chapter also introduces the concept of health, including the evolving definition of health; helps you to understand that it is the definition of health that determines the kinds of factors that are assessed; and shows you that the amount of data gathered during assessment varies with the person's age, developmental state, physical condition, risk factors, and culture.

READING ASSIGNMENT

Jarvis, *Physical Examination and Health Assessment*, 4th ed., Chapter 1. pp. 1-12.

GLOSSARY

Study the following terms after reading the corresponding chapter in the text. You should be able to cover the definition on the right and define the term out loud.

Assessment .... the collection of data about an individual's health state

Biomedical model .... the Western European/North American tradition that views health as the absence of disease

Complete data base .... a complete health history and full physical examination

Critical thinking .... simultaneously problem-solving while self-improving one's own thinking ability

Diagnostic reasoning................. a method of collecting and analyzing clinical information with the following components: 1) attending to initially available cues; 2) formulating diagnostic hypotheses; 3) gathering data relative to the tentative hypotheses; 4) evaluating each hypothesis with the new data collected, arriving at a final diagnosis

Emergency data base................. rapid collection of the data base, often compiled concurrently with life-saving measures

Environment............................ the total of all the conditions and elements that make up the surroundings and influence the development of a person

Episodic data base..................... one used for a limited or short-term problem; concerns mainly one problem, one cue complex, or one body system

Follow-up data base.................. used in all settings to monitor progress on short-term or chronic health problems

Holistic health......................... the view that the mind, body, and spirit are interdependent and function as a whole within the environment

Medical diagnosis...................... used to evaluate the cause and etiology of disease; focus is on the function or malfunction of a specific organ system

Nursing diagnosis...................... used to evaluate the response of the whole person to actual or potential health problems

Nursing process........................ a method of collecting and analyzing clinical information with the following components: 1) assessment; 2) diagnosis; 3) outcome identification; 4) planning; 5) implementation; and 6) evaluation

Objective data........................... what the health professional observes by inspecting, palpating, percussing, and auscultating during the physical examination

Prevention................................. any action directed toward promoting health and preventing the occurrence of disease

Subjective data......................... what the person says about himself or herself during history taking

Wellness................................... a dynamic process and view of health; a move toward optimal functioning

STUDY GUIDE

After completing the reading assignment, you should be able to answer the following questions in the spaces provided.

1. The steps of the diagnostic reasoning process are listed below. Consider the clinical example given for "cue recognition," and fill in the remaining diagnostic reasoning steps.

Stage	Example
Cue recognition	A.J., 62-year-old male, appears pale, diaphoretic, and anxious
Hypothesis formulation	
Data gathering for hypothesis testing	
Hypothesis evaluation	

2. One of the critical thinking skills is identifying assumptions. Explain how the following statement contains an assumption. How would you get the facts in this situation? *"Ellen, you have to break up with your boyfriend. He is too rough with you. He is no good for you."*

3. Another critical thinking skill involves validation, or checking the accuracy and reliability of data. Describe how you would validate the following data. Mr. Quinn tells you his weight this morning on the clinic scale was 165 lbs.

   The primary counselor tells you Ellen is depressed and angry about being admitted to residential treatment in the clinic.

   When auscultating the heart, you hear a blowing, swooshing sound between the first and second heart sounds.

4. Relate each of the following concepts of health to the process of data collection:

   biomedical model

   wellness

   holistic health

   health promotion and disease prevention

5. Differentiate **subjective** data from **objective** data by placing an **S** or **O** after each of the following: complaint of sore shoulder _____; unconscious _____; blood in the urine _____; family has just moved to a new area _____; dizziness _____; sore throat _____; earache _____; weight gain _____.

6. How are medical diagnosis and nursing diagnosis similar?

   How are they different?

7. For the following situations, state the type of data collection you would perform (i.e., *complete* data base, *episodic* or problem-centered data base, *follow-up* data base, *emergency* data base). Barbiturate overdose _____; ambulatory, apparently well individual who presents at outpatient clinic with a rash _____; first visit to a health care provider for a "checkup" _____; recently placed on antihypertensive medication _____.

8. Discuss the term *minority* as it applies to culturally diverse individuals.

9. List three health care interactions you have experienced yourself with another person from a culture or ethnicity different from your own. You may have been the patient or the provider—it makes no difference.

10. Using one sentence or group of phrases, how would you describe your own health state to someone you are meeting for the first time?

REVIEW QUESTIONS

This test is for you and is intended to check your own mastery of the content. Answers are provided in Appendix A.

1. The concept of health has expanded in the past 40 years. Select the phrase that reflects the most narrow description of health.

   a) the absence of disease
   b) a dynamic process toward optimal functioning
   c) depends on an interaction of mind, body, and spirit within the environment
   d) prevention of disease

2. Select the most complete description of a data base.

   a) subjective and objective data gathered by a health practitioner from a patient
   b) objective data obtained from a patient through inspection, percussion, palpation, and auscultation
   c) a summary of a patient's record, including laboratory studies
   d) subjective and objective data gathered from a patient plus the results of any diagnostic studies completed

3. Nursing diagnoses, based on assessment of a number of factors, give nurses a common language with which to communicate nursing findings. The best description of a nursing diagnosis is:

   a) used to evaluate the etiology of a disease.
   b) a pattern of coping.
   c) a concise description of actual or potential health problems or of wellness strengths.
   d) the patient's perception of and satisfaction with his or her own health status.

4. Depending on the clinical situation, the nurse may establish one of four kinds of data base. An episodic data base is described as:

   a) including a complete health history and full physical examination.
   b) concerning mainly one problem.
   c) evaluation of a previously identified problem.
   d) rapid collection of data in conjunction with lifesaving measures.

5. Individuals should be seen at regular intervals for health care. The frequency of these visits:

   a) is most efficient if performed on an annual basis.
   b) is not important. There is no recommendation for the frequency of health care.
   c) varies, depending upon the age of the person.
   d) is based on the practitioner's clinical experience.

6. Cultural diversity is currently considered when discussing health assessment and care. From a nursing perspective, the most accurate description of this phenomenon is:

   a) nursing is inherently a transcultural phenomenon. The process of helping people involves at least two people having different cultural orientations.
   b) a consideration when the nurse is caring for someone identified as a minority among the local population.
   c) the consideration of the needs of the population of the United States that does not have European ancestry.
   d) an area that has always been of consideration to nursing and is included in most nursing curricula.

CHAPTER 2

Developmental Tasks and Health Promotion Across the Life Cycle

PURPOSE

This chapter gives a general portrayal of the individual in each stage of the life cycle, considering the physical, psychosocial, cognitive, and behavioral development of the person; presents age-specific charts for periodic health examination that detail the screening examination measures, counseling for health promotion, and risk factors for each age group; and presents a few developmental screening tests used in clinical practice.

READING ASSIGNMENT

Jarvis, *Physical Examination and Health Assessment*, 4th ed., Chapter 2, pp. 13-38.

GLOSSARY

Study the following terms after reading the corresponding chapter in the text. You should be able to cover the definition on the right and define the term out loud.

Centration.................................. the characteristic of focusing on only one aspect of a situation at a time and ignoring other characteristics

Cooperative play .... children playing the same game and interacting while doing it

Delayed imitation .... a child can witness an event, form a mental representation of it, and imitate it later in the absence of the model

Egocentric .... the characteristic of focusing on one's own interests, needs, and point of view and lacking concern for others

Mental representation............... Piaget's term for the concept acquired by age 2 that an infant can think of an external event without actually experiencing it

Object permanence.................... Piaget's term for the concept acquired during infancy that objects and people continue to exist even when they are no longer in sight

Prehension............................... using the hand and fingers for the act of grasping

Stress.. the total of the biologic reactions to an adverse stimulus—whether it be physical, mental, or emotional, internal or external—that tends to disturb the homeostasis of the body

Symbolic function.................... Piaget's term for the concept acquired during childhood in which the child uses symbols to represent people, objects, and events

Telegraphic speech.................... speech used by age 3 or 4 in which three- or four-word sentences contain only the essential words

Transductive reasoning............. the young child's thinking that when two events occur simultaneously, that one caused the other, even though they are unrelated

STUDY GUIDE

After completing the reading assignment, you should be able to answer the following questions in the spaces provided.

1. List 9 developmental stages, from infancy through late adulthood, and give the general age ranges for each stage.

2. List Erikson's 8 stages of ego development that encompass the life span, and state the distinct psychological conflict that characterizes each stage.

3. List Piaget's stages of cognitive development in the growing child and state the way of thinking that characterizes each stage.

4. List at least 4 points of parent counseling that you should include on a periodic health examination for an infant, age birth to 18 months (see Table 2–1, p. 17 in Jarvis, *Physical Examination and Health Assessment*, 4th ed.).

5. Define toddler lordosis.

6. State 4 points of physical examination screening you should perform during a young child's periodic health examination, ages 2 to 6.

7. The preadolescent growth spurt occurs at about age _____ in girls and about age _____ in boys.

8. State at least 6 points of patient and parent counseling you should include during the periodic health examination for the middle childhood years, ages 7 to 12.

9. List at least 4 developmental tasks that characterize the stage of adolescence.

10. List the points of counseling for substance use, sexual practices, and injury prevention that you would include during patient teaching in the periodic health examination of an adolescent, ages 13 to 18.

11. List 5 items of physical examination aimed at screening certain high-risk groups during a periodic health examination on a younger adult.

12. State the frequency with which the following tests of physical examination should be performed on a middle-aged adult.

Clinical breast examination for women _____

Papanicolaou smear for women _____

Fecal occult blood test and/or sigmoidoscopy _____

Influenza vaccine for those at risk _____

13. State the 5 leading causes of death in older adults, ages 65 and over.

14. List the screening laboratory/diagnostic procedures that should be performed yearly on older adults, ages 65 and over.

15. Discuss the implications of conducting a life review, which is one of the developmental tasks confronting older adults.

Note that 6 tables summarizing growth and development milestones for infancy through adolescence can be found in the appendices of this Laboratory Manual, for your reference.

REVIEW QUESTIONS

This test is for you and is intended to check your own mastery of the content. Answers are provided in Appendix A.

1. Select the best description of the physical growth of an average term infant during the first year of life.

    a) between 5 and 7 pounds at birth; weight and height double by 1 year
    b) between 5½ and 10 pounds at birth; weight and height triple by 1 year
    c) between 5½ and 10 pounds at birth; weight triples and height increases 50% by 1 year
    d) 7½ pounds at birth; weight and height double by 1 year

2. Human development has been studied by a number of theorists. The best description of Erik Erikson's theory is that it is:

    a) concerned with biologic determinants of behavior.
    b) concerned with the growth of the ego.
    c) concerned with cognitive development in the growing child.
    d) concerned with physiologic development from infancy to 1 year.

3. A game of hide and seek is an example of:

    a) Piaget's object permanence.
    b) Levinson's settling down.
    c) failure to inhibit primitive reflexes.
    d) Erikson's theory of trust versus mistrust.

4. Beth D., age 15 months, has come to the clinic for a well-baby visit. This is the first visit for this child since the family recently relocated. When a developmental history is taken from the mother, she states, "Beth just started to pull herself up to a standing position." The best action on the part of the practitioner is to:

   a) proceed with the exam. The child is progressing at the expected rate.
   b) proceed with the exam. Although the child is behind the anticipated developmental stage, the child is clearly progressing in a cephalocaudal direction.
   c) perform a complete examination, focusing on the musculoskeletal system. Then discuss the findings with the mother.
   d) obtain a more detailed physical development history, then perform the examination. This represents a developmental delay for this child.

5. The use of two-word phrases by a 2-year-old is an example of:

   a) biphrase.
   b) holophrase.
   c) telegraphic speech.
   d) ritualism.

6. A group of children are observed interacting while playing the same game. The observer would recognize this as:

   a) parallel play.
   b) language development.
   c) decentration.
   d) cooperative play.

7. The description of alternative periods of structure building and transition in an adult's life are the results of the work of:

   a) Erik Erikson.
   b) National Institutes of Health.
   c) U.S. Preventive Services Task Force.
   d) Daniel Levinson.

8. A life review or a cataloging of life events is usually associated with the developmental period of:

   a) early adulthood.
   b) middle adulthood.
   c) late adulthood.
   d) grieving for the lost loved one.

9. Tabrina J. is a 17-year-old high school student who arrives for her sports physical. Which of these questions is it most appropriate to ask for counseling in prevention?

   a) How about cigarettes—do you smoke?
   b) How much milk do you drink?
   c) Have you had a flu shot this year?
   d) When was your last vision check?

10. The purpose of the Denver II screening instrument is to:

    a) provide epidemiological data.
    b) form an intelligence test.
    c) detect developmental delays.
    d) reduce risk factors.

11. Disease morbidity is increased in middle adulthood, probably caused most often by:

    a) drinking two alcoholic drinks per day.
    b) obesity.
    c) physical exertion.
    d) stress.

12. The most common age for SIDS to occur is between:

    a) birth and 2 months of age.
    b) 2 and 4 months of age.
    c) 4 and 6 months of age.
    d) 6 months and 1 year of age.

SKILLS LABORATORY/CLINICAL SETTING

You are now ready for the clinical component of mastering the content in this chapter. The purpose of the clinical component is to practice administering the developmental screening tests on a volunteer or a peer and gain some comfort with the tool before administering it on patients of your own.

The Hassles and Uplifts Scale (Table 2–1) is a tool that attempts to quantify the impact of daily life stress on an adult's health. You should take this questionnaire yourself. Be aware that some of the questions are sensitive and considered personal by many people. You should be aware of this when considering whether or not to discuss your own questionnaire with your classmate or faculty member. You will gain considerable insight in taking the test, both on the impact of daily stress on adults and on the amount of daily stress occuring in your own life.

The Denver II is a screening instrument designed to detect developmental delays in infants and preschoolers and is described in more detail in Jarvis, *Physical Examination and Health Assessment*, 4th ed., pp. 32-33. Study the text and make certain you are familiar with the tool. The Denver II was carefully standardized with very specific instructions for the administration and interpretation of each item. These are contained in the Denver II Training Manual. In addition to the instrument, you will need a kit of items (yarn, cube, doll, etc.) that are used during the test. Also, you will need a healthy young child on whom to practice. Perhaps a classmate or a faculty member can volunteer his or her young child for one administration of the test.

NOTES

TABLE 2–1. The Hassles and Uplifts Scale

HASSLES are irritants—things that annoy or bother you; they can make you upset or angry. UPLIFTS are events that make you feel good; they can make you joyful, glad, or satisfied. Some hassles and uplifts occur on a fairly regular basis and others are relatively rare. Some have only a slight effect, others have a strong effect.

This questionnaire lists things that can be hassles and uplifts in day-to-day life. You will find that during the course of a day some of these things will have been only a hassle for you and some will have been only an uplift. *Others will have been both a hassle AND an uplift.*

DIRECTIONS: Please think about how much of a hassle and how much of an uplift each item was for you today. Please indicate on the left-hand side of the page (under "HASSLES") how much of a hassle the item was by circling the appropriate number. Then indicate on the right-hand side of the page (under "UPLIFTS") how much of an uplift it was for you by circling the appropriate number.

Remember, circle one number on the left-hand side of the page *and* one number on the right-hand side of the page for *each* item.

PLEASE FILL OUT THIS QUESTIONNAIRE JUST BEFORE YOU GO TO BED.

HASSLES AND UPLIFTS SCALE

How much of a hassle was this item for you today?
HASSLES
0 = *None or not applicable*
1 = *Somewhat*
2 = *Quite a bit*
3 = *A great deal*

How much of an uplift was this item for you today?
UPLIFTS
0 = *None or not applicable*
1 = *Somewhat*
2 = *Quite a bit*
3 = *A great deal*

DIRECTIONS: Please circle one number on the left-hand side *and* one number on the right-hand side for each item.

HASSLES		UPLIFTS
0 1 2 3	1. Your child(ren)	0 1 2 3
0 1 2 3	2. Your parents or parents-in-law	0 1 2 3
0 1 2 3	3. Other relative(s)	0 1 2 3
0 1 2 3	4. Your spouse	0 1 2 3
0 1 2 3	5. Time spent with family	0 1 2 3
0 1 2 3	6. Health or well-being of a family member	0 1 2 3
0 1 2 3	7. Sex	0 1 2 3
0 1 2 3	8. Intimacy	0 1 2 3
0 1 2 3	9. Family-related obligations	0 1 2 3
0 1 2 3	10. Your friend(s)	0 1 2 3
0 1 2 3	11. Fellow workers	0 1 2 3
0 1 2 3	12. Clients, customers, patients, etc.	0 1 2 3
0 1 2 3	13. Your supervisor or employer	0 1 2 3
0 1 2 3	14. The nature of your work	0 1 2 3
0 1 2 3	15. Your work load	0 1 2 3
0 1 2 3	16. Your job security	0 1 2 3
0 1 2 3	17. Meeting deadlines or goals on the job	0 1 2 3
0 1 2 3	18. Enough money for necessities (e.g., food, clothing, housing, health care, taxes, insurance)	0 1 2 3
0 1 2 3	19. Enough money for education	0 1 2 3
0 1 2 3	20. Enough money for emergencies	0 1 2 3
0 1 2 3	21. Enough money for extras (e.g., entertainment, recreation, vacations)	0 1 2 3
0 1 2 3	22. Financial care for someone who doesn't live with you	0 1 2 3
0 1 2 3	23. Investments	0 1 2 3
0 1 2 3	24. Your smoking	0 1 2 3
0 1 2 3	25. Your drinking	0 1 2 3
0 1 2 3	26. Mood-altering drugs	0 1 2 3
0 1 2 3	27. Your physical appearance	0 1 2 3
0 1 2 3	28. Contraception	0 1 2 3
0 1 2 3	29. Exercise(s)	0 1 2 3
0 1 2 3	30. Your medical care	0 1 2 3
0 1 2 3	31. Your health	0 1 2 3
0 1 2 3	32. Your physical abilities	0 1 2 3
0 1 2 3	33. The weather	0 1 2 3
0 1 2 3	34. News events	0 1 2 3
0 1 2 3	35. Your environment (e.g., quality of air, noise level, greenery)	0 1 2 3
0 1 2 3	36. Political or social issues	0 1 2 3
0 1 2 3	37. Your neighborhood (e.g., neighbors, setting)	0 1 2 3
0 1 2 3	38. Conserving (gas, electricity, water, gasoline, etc.)	0 1 2 3
0 1 2 3	39. Pets	0 1 2 3
0 1 2 3	40. Cooking	0 1 2 3
0 1 2 3	41. Housework	0 1 2 3
0 1 2 3	42. Home repairs	0 1 2 3
0 1 2 3	43. Yardwork	0 1 2 3
0 1 2 3	44. Car maintenance	0 1 2 3
0 1 2 3	45. Taking care of paperwork (e.g., paying bills, filling out forms)	0 1 2 3
0 1 2 3	46. Home entertainment (e.g., TV, music, reading)	0 1 2 3
0 1 2 3	47. Amount of free time	0 1 2 3
0 1 2 3	48. Recreation and entertainment outside the home (e.g., movies, sports, eating out, walking)	0 1 2 3
0 1 2 3	49. Eating (at home)	0 1 2 3
0 1 2 3	50. Church or community organizations	0 1 2 3
0 1 2 3	51. Legal matters	0 1 2 3
0 1 2 3	52. Being organized	0 1 2 3
0 1 2 3	53. Social commitments	0 1 2 3

From De Longis A, Folkman S, Lazarus RS: The impact of daily stress on health and mood: Psychological and social resources as mediators. *Journal of Personality and Social Psychology* 54(3): 486–495, 1988. Copyright © 1988 by the American Psychological Association. Reprinted with permission.

Notes

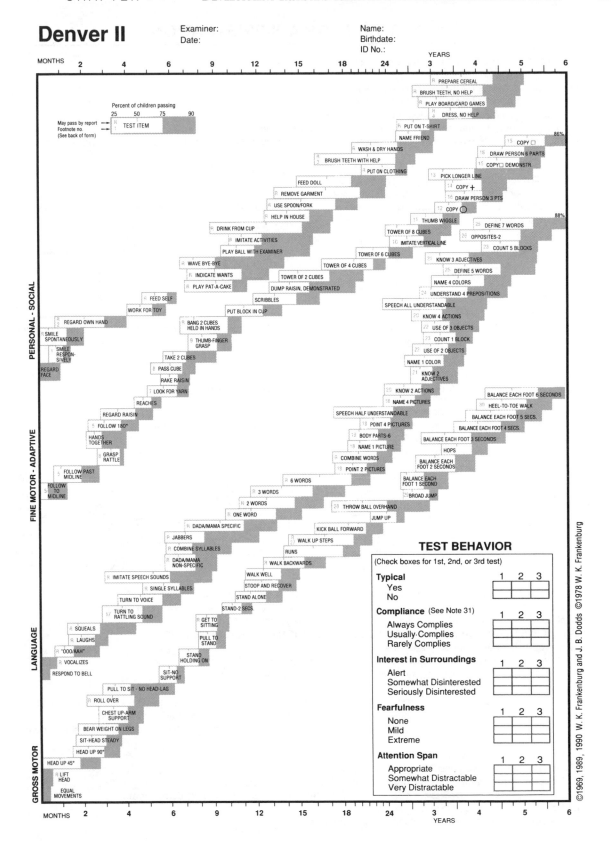

Denver II

DIRECTIONS FOR ADMINISTRATION

1. Try to get child to smile by smiling, talking or waving. Do not touch him/her.
2. Child must stare at hand several seconds.
3. Parent may help guide toothbrush and put toothpaste on brush.
4. Child does not have to be able to tie shoes or button/zip in the back.
5. Move yarn slowly in an arc from one side to the other, about 8" above child's face.
6. Pass if child grasps rattle when it is touched to the backs or tips of fingers.
7. Pass if child tries to see where yarn went. Yarn should be dropped quickly from sight from tester's hand without arm movement.
8. Child must transfer cube from hand to hand without help of body, mouth, or table.
9. Pass if child picks up raisin with any part of thumb and finger.
10. Line can vary only 30 degrees or less from tester's line. $\lor$
11. Make a fist with thumb pointing upward and wiggle only the thumb. Pass if child imitates and does not move any fingers other than the thumb.

    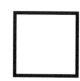

12. Pass any enclosed form. Fail continuous round motions.	13. Which line is longer? (Not bigger.) Turn paper upside down and repeat. (pass 3 of 3 or 5 of 6)	14. Pass any lines crossing near midpoint.	15. Have child copy first. If failed, demonstrate.

When giving items 12, 14, and 15, do not name the forms. Do not demonstrate 12 and 14.

16. When scoring, each pair (2 arms, 2 legs, etc.) counts as one part.
17. Place one cube in cup and shake gently near child's ear, but out of sight. Repeat for other ear.
18. Point to picture and have child name it. (No credit is given for sounds only.)
    If less than 4 pictures are named correctly, have child point to picture as each is named by tester.

19. Using doll, tell child: Show me the nose, eyes, ears, mouth, hands, feet, tummy, hair. Pass 6 of 8.
20. Using pictures, ask child: Which one flies?... says meow?... talks?... barks?... gallops? Pass 2 of 5, 4 of 5.
21. Ask child: What do you do when you are cold?... tired?... hungry? Pass 2 of 3, 3 of 3.
22. Ask child: What do you do with a cup? What is a chair used for? What is a pencil used for? Action words must be included in answers.
23. Pass if child correctly places *and* says how many blocks are on paper. (1, 5).
24. Tell child: Put block **on** table; **under** table; **in front of** me, **behind** me. Pass 4 of 4. (Do not help child by pointing, moving head or eyes.)
25. Ask child: What is a ball?... lake?... desk?... house?... banana?... curtain?... fence?... ceiling? Pass if defined in terms of use, shape, what it is made of, or general category (such as banana is fruit, not just yellow). Pass 5 of 8, 7 of 8.
26. Ask child: If a horse is big, a mouse is ___? If fire is hot, ice is ___? If the sun shines during the day, the moon shines during the ___? Pass 2 of 3.
27. Child may use wall or rail only, not person. May not crawl.
28. Child must throw ball overhand 3 feet to within arm's reach of tester.
29. Child must perform standing broad jump over width of test sheet (8 ½ inches).
30. Tell child to walk forward, ⊂◦⊃ ⊂◦⊃ ⊂◦⊃ ➤ heel within 1 inch of toe. Tester may demonstrate. Child must walk 4 consecutive steps.
31. In the second year, half of normal children are non-compliant.

OBSERVATIONS:

Transcultural Considerations in Assessment

PURPOSE

This chapter discusses the characteristics of culture, the dominant value orientation of various groups in North America, the cultural dimensions of health care, and the ways in which cultural practices affect health, illness, self care, and treatment measures. At the end of this unit, you should have increased sensitivity to the cultural dimensions of health care, and be able to perform a cultural assessment.

READING ASSIGNMENT

Jarvis, *Physical Examination and Health Assessment*, 4th ed., Chapter 3, pp. 39-50.

GLOSSARY

Study the following terms after reading the corresponding chapters in the text. You should be able to cover the definition on the right and define the term out loud.

Cultural imposition .... tendency to impose your beliefs, values, and patterns of behavior on individuals from another culture

Culture shock .... state of disorientation to a different cultural group because of its sudden strangeness, unfamiliarity, and incompatibility to person's perceptions and expectations

Ethnocentrism .... tendency to view your own way of life as the most desirable, acceptable, or best and to act superior to another culture's lifeways

Folk healer .... lay healer in the person's culture apart from the biomedical/scientific health care system

Lineal relationships .... ties with others by virtue of heredity and kinship

Norms .... rules by which human behavior is governed, which result from the cultural values held by the group

Religion .... an organized system of beliefs concerning the cause, nature, and purpose of the universe, especially a belief in God or gods

Spirituality.................................. each person's personal effort to find purpose and meaning in life

Subculture.................................. fairly large aggregates of people who have shared characteristics that are not common to all members of the culture

Values... a desirable or undesirable state of affairs, and a universal feature of all cultures

Yin/yang theory.......................... health exists when all aspects of the person are in perfect balance

STUDY GUIDE

After completing the reading assignment, you should be able to answer the following questions in the spaces provided.

1. List the 4 basic characteristics of culture.

2. Define the term *dominant value orientation* and state the 5 common human problems with respect to values.

3. List 3 perceptions of the human's relationship to nature, and describe the way each perception may influence a person's reaction to a chronic illness.

4. List 3 major ways that people can perceive the time dimension, and give examples of cultural groups who hold each focus.

5. List and define 3 ways in which people's relationships with others may be categorized.

6. List and describe 7 categories of families.

7. List and define 3 major theories on the ways in which people view the causes of illness.

8. Define the *yin/yang theory* of health and illness and relate this to different types of foods.

9. Define the *hot/cold theory* of health and illness and relate this to different types of foods and illnesses.

10. List at least 5 names for various folk healers, including the culture they represent.

11. Define the term *culture-bound syndrome*, and give examples from the African-American, Hispanic, Native American, and European-American cultures.

REVIEW QUESTIONS

This test is for you and is intended to check your own mastery of the content. Answers are provided in Appendix A.

1. C.D. is a lieutenant in the Navy. When considering culture as part of the assessment for this individual, the most obvious subculture is that of:

   a) sex.
   b) occupation.
   c) ethnicity.
   d) health-related characteristics.

2. E.A. has brought M., age 5, to the clinic for a periodic health screening. Interview reveals that E.A. is married to M.'s father, but is not the child's biological mother. The three live together. This is an example of a(n):

   a) nuclear family.
   b) extended family.
   c) blended family.
   d) single family.

3. Religion is best described as:

   a) an organized system of beliefs concerning the cause, nature, and purpose of the universe.
   b) a unique life experience and personal effort to find purpose and meaning in life.
   c) affiliation with one of the 1200 recognized religions in the United States.
   d) the following of established rituals, especially in conjunction with health-seeking behaviors.

4. Beliefs regarding causes of illness are part of a culture's view of health and illness. All of the theories listed below are discussed in the text *except*:

   a) the biomedical theory.
   b) the naturalistic theory.
   c) the bio-psycho-social disorder theory.
   d) the magico-religious theory.

5. Select the least accurate description of pain.

   a) The manifestation and management of pain are embedded in a cultural context.
   b) Pain is a universal phenomenon, therefore its expression is also universal.
   c) Pain is a highly personal experience, depending on cultural learning.
   d) The term *pain* is derived from the Greek word for penalty.

6. B.D. has been diagnosed in utero with spina bifida. This is an example of a(n):

   a) disorder associated with a genetic trait.
   b) culture-bound syndrome.
   c) environmentally caused disorder.
   d) disorder caused by nontraditional intervention during pregnancy.

SKILLS LABORATORY/CLINICAL SETTING

You are now ready for the clinical component of the transcultural chapter. The purpose of the clinical component is to collect data for a cultural assessment on a peer in the skills laboratory or on a patient in the clinical setting. Although you may not have been assigned chapters on the health history as yet, the questions in the cultural assessment tool are clearly defined and should pose no problem. The very best experience would be for you to pair up with a peer from a cultural group different from your own. If this is not possible, you still will gain insight and sensitivity into the cultural dimensions of health, and will gain mastery of the assessment tool.

CULTURAL ASSESSMENT

Brief History of the Cultural Group with which the Person Identifies (Record responses below)

- With what cultural group(s) do you affiliate (e.g., Hispanic, Polish, Navajo, or combination)? To what degree do you identify with the cultural group (e.g., "we" concept of solidarity or a fringe member)?
- What is your reported racial affiliation (e.g., black, Native American, Asian, and so on)?
- Where were you born?
- Where have you lived (country, city) and when (during what years)? Note: If a recent relocation to the United States, knowledge of prevalent diseases in country of origin may be helpful.

Values Orientation

- What are your attitudes, values, and beliefs about birth, death, health, illness, health care providers?
- How do you view work, leisure, education?
- How do you perceive change?

Cultural Sanctions and Restrictions

- How does your cultural group regard expression of emotion and feelings, spirituality, and religious beliefs? How are dying, death, and grieving expressed in a culturally appropriate manner?
- How is modesty expressed by men and women? Are there culturally defined expectations about male-female relationships, including the health care relationship?
- Do you have any restrictions related to sexuality, exposure of body parts, certain types of surgery (e.g., amputation, vasectomy, hysterectomy)?
- Are there any restrictions against discussion of dead relatives or fears related to the unknown?

Communication

- What language do you speak at home? What other languages do you speak or read? In what language would you prefer to communicate?
- Do you need an interpreter? If so, is there a relative or friend who would like to interpret? Is there anyone whom you would prefer did not interpret (e.g., member of the opposite sex, a person younger/older than you, member of a rival tribe or nation)?
- How do you feel about health care providers who are not of the same cultural background (e.g., African-American, middle-class nurse and Hispanic of a different social class)? Do you prefer to receive care from a nurse or doctor of the same cultural background, gender, and/or age?

Health-Related Beliefs and Practices

- To what cause(s) do you attribute illness and disease (e.g., divine wrath, imbalance in hot/cold or yin/yang, punishment for moral transgressions, hex, soul loss)?
- What do you believe promotes health (eating certain foods, wearing amulates to bring good luck, exercise, prayer, rituals to ancestors, saints, or intermediate deities)?
- What is your religious affiliation (e.g., Judaism, Islam, Pentecostalism, West African voodooism, Seventh-Day Adventism, Catholicism, Mormonism)?
- Do you rely on cultural healers (e.g., curandero, shaman, spiritualist, priest, minister, monk)? Who determines when you are sick and you are healthy? Who determines the type of healer and treatment that should be sought?
- In what types of cultural healing practices do you engage (use of herbal remedies, potions, massage, wearing of talismans or charms to discourage evil spirits, healing rituals, incantations, prayers)?
- How are biomedical/scientific health care providers perceived? How do you and your family perceive nurses or physicians? What are the expectations of nurses and nursing care?
- What is appropriate "sick role" behavior? Who determines what symptoms constitute disease/illness? Who decides when you are no longer sick? Who cares for you at home?
- How does your cultural group view mental disorders? Are there differences in acceptable behaviors for physical versus psychological illnesses?

Nutrition

- What is the meaning of food and eating to you? With whom do you usually eat? What types of foods are eaten? What do you define as food? What do you believe composes a "healthy" versus an "unhealthy" diet?
- How are foods prepared at home (type of food preparation, cooking oil(s) used, length of time foods are cooked, especially vegetables, amount and type of seasoning added to various foods during preparation)?

Nutrition (*Continued*)

- Do religious beliefs and practices influence your diet (e.g., amount, type, preparation or delineation of acceptable food combinations, such as kosher diets)? Do you abstain from certain foods at regular intervals, on specific dates determined by the religious calendar, or at other times?
- If your religion mandates or encourages fasting, what does the term "fast" mean (e.g., refraining from certain types or quantities of foods, eating only during certain times of the day)? For what period of time are you expected to fast?
- During fasting, do you refrain from liquids/beverages? Does your religion allow exemption from fasting during illness? If so, do you believe that an exemption applies to you?

Socioeconomic Considerations

- Who composes your social network (family, peers, and cultural healers)? How do they influence your health or illness status?
- How do members of your social support network define caring (e.g., being continuously present, doing things for you, looking after your family)? What are the roles of various family members during health and illness?
- How does your family participate in the nursing care (e.g., bathing, feeding, touching, being present)?
- Does the cultural family structure influence your response to health or illness (e.g., beliefs, strengths, weaknesses, and social class)? Is there a key family member whose role is significant in health-related decisions (e.g., grandmother in many African-American families, eldest adult son in Asian families)?
- Who is the principal wage earner in your family? What is the total annual income? (Note: This is a potentially sensitive question that should be asked only if necessary.) Is there more than one wage earner? Are there other sources of financial support (extended family, investments)?
- What impact does economic status have on lifestyle, place of residence, living conditions, ability to obtain health care, discharge planning?

Organizations Providing Cultural Support

- What influence do ethnic/cultural organizations have on your receiving health care (e.g., Organizations of Migrant Workers, National Association for the Advancement of Colored People [NAACP], Black Political Caucus, churches, schools, Urban League, community-based health care programs and clinics).

Educational Background

- What is your highest educational level obtained?
- Can you read and write English, or is another language preferred? If English is the second language, are materials available in the primary language?
- What learning style is most comfortable/familiar? Do you prefer to learn through written materials, oral explanation, or demonstration?

Religious Affiliation

- What is the role of religious beliefs and practices during health and illness?
- Are there healing rituals or practices that you believe can promote well-being or hasten recovery from illness? If so, who performs these?
- What is the role of significant religious representatives during health and illness? Are there recognized healers (e.g., Islamic imams, Christian Scientist practitioners or nurses, Catholic priests, Mormon elders, Buddhist monks)?

Spiritual Considerations

- Does the person have religious objects in the environment?
- Does the person wear outer- or undergarments having religious significance?
- Are get-well greeting cards religious in nature or from a religious representative?
- Does the person appear to pray at certain times of the day or before meals?
- Does the person make special dietary requests (e.g., kosher diet; vegetarian diet; diet free from caffeine, pork, shellfish, or other specific food items)?
- Does the person read religious magazines or books?
- Does the person mention God (Allah, Buddha, Yahweh, or a synonym), prayer, faith, or other religious topics?
- Is a request made for a visit by a member of the clergy or other religious representative?
- Is there an expression of anxiety or fear about pain, suffering, death?
- Does the person prefer to interact with others or to remain alone?

Data for spiritual considerations from Andrews MM, Hanson PA: Religion, culture, and nursing. In Boyle JS, Andrews MM (Eds). *Transcultural Concepts in Nursing Care,* 4th ed. Philadelphia, J.B. Lippincott Company, 2002.

The Interview

PURPOSE

This chapter discusses the process of communication; presents the techniques of interviewing including open-ended versus closed questions, the nine types of examiner responses, the 10 "traps" of interviewing, and nonverbal skills; and considers variations in technique that are necessary for individuals of different ages, for those with special needs, and for culturally diverse people.

READING ASSIGNMENT

Jarvis, *Physical Examination and Health Assessment*, 4th ed., Chapter 4, pp. 51-72.

AUDIO-VISUAL ASSIGNMENT

GLOSSARY

Study the following terms after reading the corresponding chapter in the text. You should be able to cover the definition on the right and define the term out loud.

Animism .... imagining that inanimate objects (e.g., a blood pressure cuff) come alive and have human characteristics

Avoidance language .... the use of euphemisms to avoid reality or to hide feelings

Clarification .... examiner's response used when the patient's word choice is ambiguous or confusing

Closed questions .... questions that ask for specific information; elicit a short, one- or two-word answer, a yes or no, or a forced choice

Confrontation .... response in which examiner gives honest feedback about what he or she has seen or felt after observing a certain patient action, feeling, or statement

Distancing.................................. the use of impersonal speech to put space between the self and a threat

Empathy .... viewing the world from the other person's inner frame of reference while remaining yourself; recognizing and accepting the other person's feelings without criticism

Ethnocentrism........................... the tendency to view your own way of life as the most desirable, acceptable, or best and to act in a superior manner to another culture's lifeways

Explanation .... examiner's statements that inform the patient; examiner shares factual and objective information

Facilitation................................. examiner's response that encourages the patient to say more, to continue with the story

Interpretation .... examiner's statement that is not based on direct observation, but is based on examiner's inference or conclusion; it links events, makes associations, or implies cause

Interview.................................... meeting between examiner and patient with the goal of gathering a complete health history

Jargon .... using medical vocabulary with patient in an exclusionary and paternalistic way

Leading question .... a question that implies that one answer would be better than another

Nonverbal communication ...... message conveyed through body language—posture, gestures, facial expression, eye contact, touch, and even where one places the chairs

Open-ended questions.............. asks for longer narrative information; unbiased; leaves the person free to answer in any way

Reflection.................................. examiner response that echoes the patient's words; repeats part of what patient has just said

Summary.................................... final review of what examiner understands patient has said; condenses facts and presents a survey of how the examiner perceives the health problem or need

Verbal communication .... messages sent through spoken words, vocalizations, tone of voice

STUDY GUIDE

After completing the reading assignment and the audio-visual assignment, you should be able to answer the following questions in the spaces provided.

1. List 8 items of information that should be communicated to the patient concerning the terms or expectations of the interview.

2. Describe the points to consider in preparing the physical setting for the interview.

3. List the pros and cons of note-taking during the interview.

4. Contrast open-ended versus closed questions and explain the purpose of each during the interview.

5. List the 9 types of examiner responses that could be used during the interview, and give a short example of each.

6. List the 10 traps of interviewing, and give a short example of each.

7. State at least 7 types of nonverbal behaviors that an interviewer could make.

8. State a useful phrase to use as a closing when ending the interview.

9. Discuss special considerations when interviewing the older adult.

10. Discuss ways you would modify your interviewing technique when working with a hearing-impaired person.

11. Formulate a response you would make to a patient who has spoken to you in ways you interpret as sexually aggressive.

12. Discuss the ways that nonverbal behavior may vary cross-culturally.

13. List at least 5 points to consider when using an interpreter during an interview.

REVIEW QUESTIONS

This test is for you and is intended to check your own mastery of the content. Answers are provided in Appendix A.

1. The practitioner, entering the examining room to meet a patient for the first time, states: "Hello, I'm M.M., and I'm here to gather some information from you and to perform your examination. This will take about 30 minutes. D.D. is a student working with me. If it's all right with you, she will remain during the examination." Which of the following must be added in order to cover all aspects of the interview contract?

   a) a statement regarding confidentiality, patient costs, and the expectation of each person
   b) the purpose of the interview and the role of the examiner
   c) time and place of the interview and a confidentiality statement
   d) an explicit purpose of the interview and a description of the physical examination, including diagnostic studies

2. An accurate understanding of the other person's feelings within a communication context is an example of:

   a) empathy.
   b) liking others.
   c) facilitation.
   d) a nonverbal listening technique.

3. You have come into a patient's room to conduct an admission interview. Because you are expecting a phone call, you stand near the door during the interview. A more appropriate approach would be to:

   a) arrange to have someone page you so you can sit on the side of the bed.
   b) have someone else answer the phone so you can sit facing the patient.
   c) use this approach given the circumstances; it is correct.
   d) arrange for a time free of interruptions until the initial physical examination is complete.

4. Students frequently ask teachers, "May I ask you a question?" This is an example of:

   a) an open-ended question.
   b) a reflective question.
   c) a closed question.
   d) a double-barreled question.

5. During a patient interview, you recognize the need to use interpretation. This verbal response:

   a) is the same as clarification.
   b) is a summary of a statement made by a patient.
   c) is used to focus on a particular aspect of what the patient has just said.
   d) is based on the interviewer's inference from the data that have been presented.

6. A good rule for an interviewer is to:

   a) stop the patient each time something is said that is not understood.
   b) spend more time listening to the patient than talking.
   c) consistently think of your next response so the patient will know you understand him.
   d) use "why" questions to seek clarification of unusual symptoms or behavior.

7. During an interview, a patient denies having any anxiety. The patient frequently changes position in the chair, holds his arms folded tight against his chest, and has little eye contact with the interviewer. The interviewer should:

    a) use confrontation to bring the discrepancy between verbal and nonverbal behavior to the patient's attention.
    b) proceed with the interview. Patients usually are truthful with a health care practitioner.
    c) make a mental note to discuss the behavior after the physical examination is completed.
    d) proceed with the interview and exam as outlined on the agency assessment form. The patient's behavior is appropriate for the circumstances.

8. Touch should be used during the interview:

    a) only with individuals from a Western culture.
    b) as a way of establishing contact with the person and communicating empathy.
    c) only with patients of the same sex.
    d) only if the interviewer knows the person well.

9. Children are usually brought for health care by a parent. At about what age should the interviewer begin to question the child him- or herself regarding presenting symptoms?

    a) 5
    b) 7
    c) 9
    d) 11

10. Because of adolescents' developmental level, not all interviewing techniques can be used with them. The two to be avoided are:

    a) facilitation and clarification.
    b) confrontation and explanation.
    c) empathy and interpretations.
    d) silence and reflection.

11. Knowledge of the use of personal space is helpful for the health care provider. Personal distance is generally considered to be:

    a) 0 to 1½ feet.
    b) 1½ to 4 feet.
    c) 4 to 12 feet.
    d) 12 or more feet.

12. Mr. B. tells you, "Everyone here ignores me." You respond, "Ignores you?" This technique is best described as:

    a) clarification.
    b) selective listening.
    c) reflecting.
    d) validation.

13. Active listening skills include all of the following *except*:

    a) taking detailed notes during the interview.
    b) watching for clues in body language.
    c) repeating statements back to the person to make sure you have understood.
    d) asking open-ended questions to explore the person's perspective.
    e) exploring the person's fears about his or her illness.

Note that the clinical component of this chapter is the gathering of the complete health history. The history forms are included in Chapter 6.

Domestic Violence Assessment

PURPOSE

This chapter helps you learn about intimate partner violence and elder abuse, including how to assess the extent of the abuse, the extent of physical and psychological harm, including injury, and how to document appropriately.

READING ASSIGNMENT

Jarvis, *Physical Examination and Health Assessment*, 4th ed., Chapter 5, pp. 73-82.

GLOSSARY

Study the following terms after reading the corresponding chapter in the text. You should be able to cover the definition on the right and define the term out loud.

Elder abuse .... willful infliction of force that results in bodily harm, pain, and/or impairment on a person age 65 or older. Examples include pushing, slapping, hitting, shaking, burning, and rough handling.

Elder neglect (physical) .... physical harm (actual or potential) to person age 65 or older because of failure to provide for the person's well-being. Examples include inadequate feeding and hydration, unsanitary living conditions, and poor personal hygiene.

Intimate partner violence (IPV) .... physical and/or sexual violence (use of physical force) or threat of such violence; also psychological/emotional abuse and/or coercive tactics when there has been prior physical and/or sexual violence between persons who are spouses or nonmarital partners (dating, boyfriend-girlfriend) or former spouses or nonmarital partners.

Mandatory reporting of abuse .... a specified group of persons (e.g., health care providers) is required by law to report abuse (of a specified nature against specified persons) to a governmental agency (e.g., protective services, the police).

Psychological abuse .... infliction of emotional/mental anguish by humiliation, coercion, and threats and/or lack of social stimulation. Examples include yelling, threats of harm, threats of withholding basic medical and/or personal care, and leaving the person alone for long periods of time.

Routine, universal screening for intimate partner violence .... asking all adult patients (usually female patients) whether they have experienced IPV each time they are in the health care system no matter what their complaint.

STUDY GUIDE

After completing the reading assignment and the audio-visual assignment, you should be able to answer the following questions in the spaces provided.

1. Identify the most common physical health problems that result from intimate partner violence.

2. Identify the most common mental health problems that result from intimate partner violence.

3. Differentiate abuse from neglect.

4. Identify commonly used screening questions for intimate partner violence.

5. Identify commonly used screening questions for elder abuse.

6. Differentiate routine, universal screening from indicator-based screening.

7. Identify important elements of assessment for an abused person.

8. List two potential sources of lethality in intimate partner violence situations.

ADDITIONAL LEARNING ACTIVITIES

1. Read your daily newspaper for a month, cutting out stories that are related to intimate partner (domestic) violence or elder abuse, including stories about intimate partner or elder homicide. Notice details of the story, including if there is subtle "victim blaming" or various myths about abuse that are apparent.

2. Notice whether or not you were asked about intimate partner violence at your last encounter as a patient in the health care system. Check to see if your health care provider has any posters about domestic violence or brochures in the rest rooms or other accessible areas.

3. Visit your local shelter for domestic violence. Take note of what health care services are offered to women and children who are staying there. Take note of volunteer opportunities and tell your friends about them.

4. Visit your local adult protective services office. Find out what happens when a nurse makes a report about elder abuse.

5. Find out what your state laws are about mandatory reporting of intimate partner violence and elder abuse. See if your clinical practice site has policies and procedures that match the state law.

REVIEW QUESTIONS

This test is for you and is intended to check your own mastery of the content. Answers are provided in Appendix A.

1. Which of the following are examples of intimate partner violence?

   a) an ex-boyfriend stalks his ex-girlfriend
   b) marital rape
   c) hitting a date
   d) all of the above

2. Routine, universal screening for domestic violence means:

   a) asking all women who come to the health care system if they are abused each time they come.
   b) asking women who have injuries if they are abused.
   c) asking women who have symptoms of depression and PTSD if they are abused.
   d) asking women aged 18–30 if they are abused.

3. Mental health problems associated with intimate partner violence include:

   a) hallucinations.
   b) suicidality.
   c) schizophrenia.
   d) attention deficit hyperactivity disorder (ADHD).

4. Gynecological problems *not* associated with intimate partner violence include:

   a) pelvic pain.
   b) ovarian cysts.
   c) STDs.
   d) vaginal tearing.

5. Risk factors for intimate partner homicide include:

   a) abuse during pregnancy.
   b) victim substance abuse.
   c) victim unemployment.
   d) history of victim childhood sexual assault.

6. Elder abuse and neglect include:

   a) willful infliction of force.
   b) withholding prescription medications without medical orders.
   c) not replacing broken eyeglasses.
   d) threatening to place someone in a nursing home.
   e) all of the above.

CHAPTER

The Complete Health History

PURPOSE

This chapter helps you to learn the elements of a complete health history, to interview a patient to gather the data for a complete health history, to analyze the patient data, and to record the history accurately.

READING ASSIGNMENT

Jarvis, *Physical Examination and Health Assessment*, 4th ed., Chapter 6, pp. 83-104.

STUDY GUIDE

After completing the reading assignment, you should be able to answer the following questions in the spaces provided.

1. State the purpose of the complete health history.

2. List and define the critical characteristics used to explore each symptom the patient identifies.

3. Define the elements of the health history: reason for seeking care; present health state or present illness; past history, family history; review of systems; functional patterns of living.

4. Discuss the rationale for obtaining a family history.

5. Discuss the rationale for obtaining a systems review.

6. Describe the items included in a functional assessment.

7. Describe the additions/modifications you would make in environment, pacing, and content when conducting a health history on an older adult.

REVIEW QUESTIONS

This test is for you and is intended to check your own mastery of the content. Answers are provided in Appendix A.

1. When reading a medical record you see the following notation: Patient states, "I have had a cold for about a week, and now I am having difficulty breathing." This is an example of:

   a) past history.
   b) a review of systems.
   c) a functional assessment.
   d) a reason for seeking care.

2. You have reason to question the reliability of the information being provided by a patient. One way to verify the reliability within the context of the interview is to:

   a) rephrase the same questions later in the interview.
   b) review the patient's previous medical records.
   c) call the person identified as emergency contact to verify data provided.
   d) provide the patient with a printed history to complete and then compare the data provided.

3. The statement "Reason for seeking care" has replaced the "chief complaint." This change is significant because:

   a) "chief complaint" is really a diagnostic statement.
   b) the newer term allows another individual to supply the necessary information.
   c) the newer term incorporates wellness needs.
   d) "Reason for seeking care" can incorporate the history of present illness.

4. During an initial interview, the examiner asks, "Mrs. J., tell me what you do when your headaches occur." With this question, the examiner is seeking information about:

   a) the patient's perception of the problem.
   b) aggravating or relieving factors.
   c) the frequency of the problem.
   d) the severity of the problem.

5. Which of the following is an appropriate recording of a patient's reason for seeking health care?

   a) angina pectoris, duration 2 hr
   b) substernal pain radiating to left axilla, 1 hr duration
   c) "grabbing" chest pain for 2 hr
   d) pleurisy, 2 days' duration

6. A genogram is useful in showing information concisely. It is used specifically for:

   a) past history.
   b) past health history, specifically hospitalizations.
   c) family history.
   d) the eight characteristics of presenting symptoms.

7. Select the best description of "review of systems" as part of the health history.

   a) the evaluation of the past and present health state of each body system
   b) a documentation of the problem as described by the patient
   c) the recording of the objective findings of the practitioner
   d) a statement that describes the overall health state of the patient

8. Which of the following is considered to be subjective?

   a) temperature of 101.2° F
   b) pulse rate of 96
   c) measured weight loss of 20 pounds since the previous measurement
   d) pain lasting 2 hours

9. When taking a health history for a child, what information, in addition to that for an adult, is usually obtained?

   a) coping and stress management
   b) a review of immunizations received
   c) environmental hazards
   d) hospitalization history

10. Functional assessment measures how a person manages day-to-day activities. The impact of a disease on the daily activities of older adults is referred to as:

    a) interpersonal relationship assessment.
    b) instrumental activities of daily living.
    c) reason for seeking care.
    d) disease burden.

SKILLS LABORATORY/CLINICAL SETTING

You are now ready for the clinical component of the interview and health history chapters. The purpose of the clinical component is to practice conducting a complete health history on a peer in the skills laboratory and to achieve the following.

CLINICAL OBJECTIVES

1. Demonstrate knowledge of interviewing skills by: arranging a private, quiet, comfortable setting; introducing yourself and stating your goals for the interview; posing open-ended and direct questions appropriately; listening to the patient in an attentive, nonjudgmental manner; choosing appropriate vocabulary that the patient understands.

2. Demonstrate knowledge of the components of a health history by: recording the reason for seeking care in the person's own words; eliciting all the critical characteristics to describe the patient's symptom(s); gathering pertinent data for the past history, family history, and systems review; identifying self-care behaviors and risk factors from the functional assessment.

3. Record the history data accurately and as a reflection of what the patient believes the true health state to be.

INSTRUCTIONS

Work in pairs and obtain a complete health history from a peer. Although you already know each other as student colleagues, play your role straight as examiner or patient for the best learning experience. Be aware that some of the history questions cover personal content. When you are acting as the patient, you have the right to withhold an answer if you do not feel comfortable with the amount of material you will be asked to divulge. Your own rights to privacy must coexist with the goals of the learning experience.

Familiarize yourself with the following history form and practice phrasing your questions ahead of time. Note that the language on this form is intended as a prompt for the examiner and must be translated into clear and appropriate phrases for the patient. As a beginning examiner, you will need to use one copy of the form as a worksheet during the actual interview and use a fresh copy of the form for your rewritten formal record.

WRITE-UP—HEALTH HISTORY

Date _____

Examiner _____

1. Biographical Data

Name _____ Phone _____

Address _____

Birth date _____ Birthplace _____

Age _____ Sex _____ Marital Status _____ Occupation _____

Race/ethnic origin _____ Employer _____

2. Source and Reliability

3. Reason for Seeking Care

4. Present Health or History of Present Illness

5. Past Health

General Health _____

Childhood Illnesses _____

_____

Accidents or Injuries _____

_____

Serious or Chronic Illnesses _____

_____

Hospitalizations _____

_____

Operations _____

_____

Jarvis, Carolyn: PHYSICAL EXAMINATION AND HEALTH ASSESSMENT, Fourth Edition,
Student Laboratory Manual. Copyright © 2004, 2000, 1996, Elsevier Inc. All rights reserved.

Obstetric History

Gravida _____ Term _____ Preterm _____
(# pregnancies)   (# Term pregnancies) (# Preterm pregnancies)

Ab/incomplete _____ Children living _____
(# Abortions/Miscarriages)

Course of pregnancy _____
(Date delivery, length of pregnancy, length of labor, baby's weight and sex, vaginal delivery/cesarean section, complications, baby's condition)

Immunizations _____

Last examination date _____

Allergies _____ Reaction _____

Current medications _____

_____

6. Family History

Specify: Construct genogram here.

Heart disease _____

High blood pressure _____

Stroke _____

Diabetes _____

Blood disorders _____

Breast cancer _____

Cancer (other) _____

Sickle cell _____

Arthritis _____

Allergies _____

Asthma _____

Obesity _____

Alcoholism _____

Mental illness _____

Seizure disorder _____

Kidney disease _____

Tuberculosis _____

7. Review of Systems

(Include both past health problems that have been resolved and current problems, including date of onset.)

   (Circle if present.)   (Comment, if needed.)

General Overall Health State: Present weight (gain or loss, period of time, by diet or other factors), fatigue, weakness or malaise, fever, chills, sweats or night sweats.

Skin: History of skin disease (eczema, psoriasis, hives), pigment or color change, change in mole, excessive dryness or moisture, pruritus, excessive bruising, rash, or lesion.

Hair: Recent loss, change in texture.

Nails: Change in shape, color, or brittleness.
   Health Promotion: Amount of sun exposure, method of self-care for skin and hair.

Head: Any unusually frequent or severe headache, any head injury, dizziness (syncope), or vertigo.

Eyes: Difficulty with vision (decreased acuity, blurring, blind spots), eye pain, diplopia (double vision), redness or swelling, watering or discharge, glaucoma or cataracts.
   Health Promotion: Wears glasses or contacts; last vision check or glaucoma test; how coping with loss of vision if any.

Ears: Earaches, infections, discharge and its characteristics, tinnitus, or vertigo.
   Health Promotion: Hearing loss, hearing aid use, how loss affects daily life, any exposure to environmental noise, method of cleaning ears.

Nose and Sinuses: Discharge and its characteristics, any unusually frequent or severe colds, sinus pain, nasal obstruction, nosebleeds, allergies or hay fever, or change in sense of smell.

Mouth and Throat: Mouth pain, frequent sore throat, bleeding gums, toothache, lesion in mouth or tongue, dysphagia, hoarseness or voice change, tonsillectomy, altered taste.
   Health Promotion: Pattern of daily dental care, use of prostheses (dentures, bridge) and last dental checkup.

Neck: Pain, limitation of motion, lumps or swelling, enlarged or tender nodes, goiter.

Breast: Pain, lump, nipple discharge, rash, history of breast disease, any surgery on breasts.
   Axilla: Tenderness, lump or swelling, rash.
   Health Promotion: Performs breast self-examination, including its frequency and method used, last mammogram and results.

(Circle if present.)   (Comment, if needed.)

Respiratory System: History of lung disease (asthma, emphysema, bronchitis, pneumonia, tuberculosis), chest pain with breathing, wheezing or noisy breathing, shortness of breath, how much activity produces shortness of breath, cough, sputum (color, amount), hemoptysis, toxin or pollution exposure.
    Health Promotion: Last chest x-ray.

Cardiovascular System: Precordial or retrosternal pain, palpitation, cyanosis, dyspnea on exertion (specify amount of exertion it takes to produce dyspnea), orthopnea, paroxysmal nocturnal dyspnea, nocturia, edema, history of heart murmur, hypertension, coronary artery disease, anemia.
    Health Promotion: Date of last ECG or other heart tests and results.

Peripheral Vascular System: Coldness, numbness and tingling, swelling of legs (time of day, activity), discoloration in hands or feet (bluish red, pallor, mottling, associated with position, especially around feet and ankles), varicose veins or complications, intermittent claudication, thrombophlebitis, ulcers.
    Health Promotion: Does work involve long-term sitting or standing, avoid crossing legs at the knees, wear support hose.

Gastrointestinal System: Appetite, food intolerance, dysphagia, heartburn, indigestion, pain (associated with eating), other abdominal pain, pyrosis (esophageal and stomach burning sensation with sour eructation), nausea and vomiting (character), vomiting blood, history of abdominal disease (ulcer, liver or gallbladder, jaundice, appendicitis, colitis), flatulence, frequency of bowel movement, any recent change, stool characteristics, constipation or diarrhea, black stools, rectal bleeding, rectal conditions, hemorrhoids, fistula).
    Health Promotion: Use of antacids or laxatives.

Urinary System: Frequency, urgency, nocturia (the number of times the person awakens at night to urinate, recent change), dysuria, polyuria or oliguria, hesitancy or straining, narrowed stream, urine color (cloudy or presence of hematuria), incontinence, history of urinary disease (kidney disease, kidney stones, urinary tract infections, prostate), pain in flank, groin, suprapubic region, or low back.
    Health Promotion: Measures to avoid or treat urinary tract infections, use of Kegel exercises after childbirth.

Male Genital System: Penis or testicular pain, sores or lesions, penile discharge, lumps, hernia.
    Health Promotion: Perform testicular self-examination? How frequently?

Female Genital System: Menstrual history (age at menarche, last menstrual period, cycle and duration, any amenorrhea or menorrhagia, premenstrual pain or dysmenorrhea, intermenstrual spotting), vaginal itching, discharge and its characteristics, age at menopause, menopausal signs or symptoms, postmenopausal bleeding.
    Health Promotion: Last gynecologic checkup, last Pap smear and results.

(Circle if present.)   (Comment, if needed.)

Sexual Health: Presently in a relationship involving intercourse? Are aspects of sex satisfactory to you and partner, any dyspareunia (for female), any changes in erection or ejaculation (for male), use of contraceptive, is contraceptive method satisfactory? Use of condoms, how frequently? Aware of any contact with partner who has sexually transmitted disease (gonorrhea, herpes, chlamydia, venereal warts, HIV/AIDS, syphilis)?

Musculoskeletal System: History of arthritis or gout. In the joints: pain, stiffness, swelling (location, migratory nature), deformity, limitation of motion, noise with joint motion. In the muscles: any pain, cramps, weakness, gait problems or problems with coordinated activities. In the back: any pain (location and radiation to extremities), stiffness, limitation of motion, or history of back pain or disc disease.

   Health Promotion: How much walking per day. What is the effect of limited range of motion on daily activities, such as on grooming, feeding, toileting, dressing? Any mobility aids used.

Neurologic System: History of seizure disorder, stroke, fainting, blackouts. In motor function: weakness, tic or tremor, paralysis, or coordination problems. In sensory function: numbness and tingling (paresthesia). In cognitive function: memory disorder (recent or distant, disorientation). In mental status: any nervousness, mood change, depression, or any history of mental health dysfunction or hallucinations.

Hematologic System: Bleeding tendency of skin or mucous membranes, excessive bruising, lymph node swelling, exposure to toxic agents or radiation, blood transfusion and reactions.

Endocrine System: History of diabetes or diabetic symptoms (polyuria, polydipsia, polyphagia), history of thyroid disease, intolerance to heat or cold, change in skin pigmentation or texture, excessive sweating, relationship between appetite and weight, abnormal hair distribution, nervousness, tremors, and need for hormone therapy.

FUNCTIONAL ASSESSMENT (Including Activities of Daily Living)

Self-Esteem, Self-Concept: Education (last grade completed, other significant training) _____

_____

Financial status (income adequate for lifestyle and/or health concerns) _____

_____

Value-belief system (religious practices and perception of personal strengths) _____

_____

Self-care behaviors _____

_____

Activity/Exercise: Daily profile, usual pattern of a typical day _____

_____

Independent or needs assistance with ADLs, feeding, bathing, hygiene, dressing, toileting, bed-to-chair
transfer, walking, standing, climbing stairs _____

_____

Leisure activities _____

Exercise pattern (type, amount per day or week, method of warm-up session, method of monitoring
body's response to exercise) _____

_____

Other self-care behaviors _____

Sleep/Rest: Sleep patterns, daytime naps, any sleep aids used _____

_____

Other self-care behavior _____

Nutrition/Elimination: Record 24-hour diet recall _____

_____

_____

Is this menu pattern typical of most days? _____

Who buys food?_____Who prepares food? _____

Finances adequate for food?_____

Who is present at mealtimes? _____

Other self-care behaviors_____

Interpersonal Relationships/Resources:

Describe own role in family _____

How getting along with family, friends, coworkers, classmates _____

_____

Get support with a problem from _____

How much daily time spent alone? _____

Is this pleasurable or isolating?_____

Other self-care behaviors _____

Coping and Stress Management: Describe stresses in life now _____

_____

Change in past year _____

Methods used to relieve stress _____

Are these methods helpful? _____

Personal Habits: Daily intake caffeine (coffee, tea, colas) _____

_____

Smoke cigarettes? _____ Number packs per day_____

Daily use for how many years _____ Age started _____

Ever tried to quit? _____ How did it go? _____

Drink alcohol? _____ Date last alcohol use _____

Amount of alcohol that episode _____

Out of last 30 days, on how many days had alcohol? _____

Ever had a drinking problem? _____

Any use of street drugs_____

Specifically, marijuana? _____ cocaine? _____

crack cocaine? _____ amphetamines?_____

barbiturates? _____ LSD? _____

heroin? _____ other? _____

Ever been in treatment for drugs or alcohol? _____

Environment/Hazards: Housing and neighborhood (type of structure, live alone, know neighbors) _____

_____

Safety of area _____

Adequate heat and utilities _____

Access to transportation _____

Involvement in community services _____ _____

Hazards at workplace or home _____

Use of seat belts _____

Travel or residence in other countries _____

Military service in other countries _____

Self-care behaviors _____

Intimate Partner Violence: How are things at home? Do you feel safe?

_____

Ever been emotionally or physically abused by your partner or someone important to you?_____

Ever been hit, slapped, kicked, pushed or shoved, or otherwise physically hurt by your partner or ex-partner? _____

Partner ever force you into having sex? _____

Are you afraid of your partner or ex-partner? _____

Occupational Health: Please describe your job _____

Work with any health hazards (e.g., asbestos, inhalants, chemicals, repetitive motion) _____

Any equipment at work designed to reduce your exposure? _____

Any work programs designed to monitor your exposure? _____

Any health problems that you think are related to your job? _____

What do you like or dislike about your job? _____

Perception of Own Health: How do you define health? _____

View of own health now _____

What are your concerns? _____

What do you expect will happen to your health in future? _____

_____

Your health goals _____

Your expectations of nurses, physicians _____

_____

CHAPTER 7

Mental Status Assessment

PURPOSE

This chapter helps you to learn the components of the mental status examination, including assessing a person's appearance, behavior, cognitive functions, and thought processes and perceptions; to understand the rationale and methods of examination of mental status; and to record the assessment accurately.

READING ASSIGNMENT

Jarvis, *Physical Examination and Health Assessment,* 4th ed., Chapter 7, pp. 105-130.

GLOSSARY

Study the following terms after completing the reading assignment. You should be able to cover the definition on the right and define the term out loud.

Abstract reasoning .... pondering a deeper meaning beyond the concrete and literal

Attention .... concentration, ability to focus on one specific thing

Consciousness .... being aware of one's own existence, feelings, and thoughts and being aware of the environment

Language .... using the voice to communicate one's thoughts and feelings

Memory .... ability to lay down and store experiences and perceptions for later recall

Mood .... prolonged display of a person's feelings

Orientation .... awareness of the objective world in relation to the self

Perceptions .... awareness of objects through any of the five senses

Thought content .... *what* the person thinks—specific ideas, beliefs, the use of words

Thought process .... the *way* a person thinks, the logical train of thought

STUDY GUIDE

After completing the reading assignment, you should be able to answer the following questions in the spaces provided.

1. Define the term *mental disorder.*

2. List 4 situations in which it would be necessary to perform a complete mental status examination.

3. Explain 4 factors that could affect the patient's response to the mental status examination but have nothing to do with mental disorders.

4. Distinguish *dysphonia* from *dysarthria.*

5. Define *unilateral neglect,* and state the illness with which it is associated.

6. State convenient ways to assess a person's recent memory within the context of the initial health history.

7. Which mental function is the Four Unrelated Words Test intended to test?

8. List at least 3 questions you could ask a patient that would screen for suicide ideation.

9. Describe the patient response level of consciousness that would be graded as:

Lethargic or somnolent _____

Obtunded _____

Stupor or semi-coma _____

Coma _____

Delirium _____

10. State the symptoms and physical signs that are characteristic of alcohol withdrawal.

REVIEW QUESTIONS

This test is for you and is intended to check your own mastery of the content. Answers are provided in Appendix A.

1. Although a full mental status examination may not be required, the examiner must be aware of the four main headings of the assessment while performing the interview and physical examination. These headings are:

a) mood, affect, consciousness, and orientation.
b) memory, attention, thought content, and perceptions.
c) language, orientation, attention, and abstract reasoning.
d) appearance, behavior, cognition, and thought processes.

2. Select the finding that most accurately describes the appearance of a patient.

a) Tense posture and restless activity. Clothing clean but not appropriate for season; patient wearing T-shirt and shorts in cold weather.
b) Oriented × 3. Affect appropriate for circumstances.
c) Alert and responds to verbal stimuli. Tearful when diagnosis discussed.
d) Laughing inappropriately, oriented × 3.

3. The ability to lay down new memories is part of the assessment of cognitive functions. One way to accomplish this is by:

   a) noting whether the patient completes a thought without wandering.
   b) a test of general knowledge.
   c) a description of past medical history.
   d) use of the Four Unrelated Words Test.

4. In order to accurately plan for discharge teaching, additional assessments may be required for the patient with aphasia. This may be accomplished by asking the patient to:

   a) calculate serial 7s.
   b) name his or her grandchildren and their birthdays.
   c) demonstrate word comprehension by naming articles in the room or on the body as you point to them.
   d) interpret a proverb.

5. During an interview with a patient newly diagnosed with a seizure disorder, the patient states, "I plan to be an airline pilot." If the patient continues to have this as a career goal after teaching regarding seizure disorders has been provided, the practitioner might question the patient's:

   a) thought processes.
   b) judgment.
   c) attention span.
   d) recent memory.

6. On a patient's second day in an acute care hospital, the patient complains about the "bugs" on the bed. The bed is clean. This would be an example of altered:

   a) thought process.
   b) orientation.
   c) perception.
   d) higher intellectual function.

7. One way to assess cognitive function and to detect dementia is with:

   a) the Proverb Interpretation Test.
   b) the Mini-Mental State Examination.
   c) the Four Unrelated Words Test.
   d) the Older Adult Behavioral Checklist.

8. The Behavioral Checklist, completed by a parent, is used to assess the mental status of:

   a) infants.
   b) children 1 to 5 years of age.
   c) children 7 to 11 years of age.
   d) adolescents.

9. A major characteristic of dementia is:

   a) impairment of short- and long-term memory.
   b) hallucinations.
   c) sudden onset of symptoms.
   d) substance-induced.

Match column B with column A.

Column A—Definition	Column B—Type of mood and affect
10. _____ Lack of emotional response	a) Depression
11. _____ Loss of identity	b) Anxiety
12. _____ Excessive well-being	c) Flat affect
13. _____ Apprehensive from the anticipation of a danger whose source is unknown	d) Euphoria
	e) Lability
14. _____ Annoyed, easily provoked	f) Rage
15. _____ Loss of control	g) Irritability
16. _____ Sad, gloomy, dejected	h) Fear
17. _____ Rapid shift of emotions	i) Depersonalization
18. _____ Worried about known external danger	

19. Write a narrative account of a mental status assessment with normal findings.

SKILLS LABORATORY/CLINICAL SETTING

You are now ready for the clinical component of the mental status examination. The purpose of the clinical component is to achieve beginning competency with the administration of the mental status examination and with the supplemental "Mini-Mental State" examination.

Practice the steps of the full mental status examination on a peer or a patient in the clinical setting, giving appropriate instructions as you proceed. Formulate ahead of time your questions to pose to the patient. Record your findings using the regional write up sheet that follows.

Next, practice the steps of the Mini-Mental State examination, which is a simplified scored form of the cognitive functions found on the full mental status examination. It is used frequently in clinical and research settings.

NOTES

REGIONAL WRITE-UP—MENTAL STATUS EXAMINATION

Date _____

Patient _____ Age _____ Sex _____ Occupation _____

Examiner _____

Mental Status

(Before testing, tell the person the four words you want him or her to remember and to recall in a few minutes, for the Four Unrelated Words Test.)

1. Appearance

    Posture _____
    Body movements _____
    Dress _____
    Grooming and hygiene _____

2. Behavior

    Level of consciousness _____
    Facial expression _____
    Speech:
        Quality _____
        Pace _____
        Word choice _____
    Mood and affect _____

3. Cognitive Functions

    Orientation:
        Time _____
        Place _____
        Person _____
    Attention span _____
    Recent memory _____
    Remote memory _____
    New learning—Four Unrelated Words Test _____
    Additional testing for aphasia:
        Word comprehension _____
        Reading _____
        Writing _____
    Judgment _____

4. Thought Processes and Perceptions

    Thought processes _____
    Thought content _____
    Perceptions _____
    Suicidal thoughts _____

Notes

MINI-MENTAL STATE EXAMINATION (MMSE)

Sample Items

Orientation to Time
"What is the date?"

Registration
"Listen carefully, I am going to say three words. You say them back after I stop. Ready? Here they are...
HOUSE (pause), CAR (pause), LAKE (pause). Now repeat those words back to me." [Repeat up to 5 times, but score only the first trial.]

Naming
"What is this?" [Point to a pencil or pen.]

Reading
"Please read this and do what it says." [Show examinee the words on the stimulus form.]

(For a full copy of the Mini-Mental State Examination, please see page 104 in Jarvis, *Physical Examination and Health Assessment,* 4th edition.)

Nutritional Assessment

PURPOSE

This chapter helps you to learn the components of nutritional assessment, including the assessment of dietary intake and nutritional status of individuals; to identify the possible occurrence, nature, and extent of impaired nutritional status (ranging from undernutrition to overnutrition), and to record the assessment accurately.

READING ASSIGNMENT

Jarvis, *Physical Examination and Health Assessment*, 4th ed., Chapter 8. pp. 131-160.

GLOSSARY

Study the following terms after completing the reading assignment. You should be able to cover the definition on the right and define the term out loud.

Android obesity .... excess body fat that is placed predominantly within the abdomen and upper body, as opposed to the hips and thighs

Anergy .... a less-than-expected or absent immune reaction in response to the injection of antigens within the skin

Anthropometry .... measurement of the body, e.g., height, weight, circumferences, skinfold thickness

Body mass index .... Weight in kilograms divided by height in meters squared (W/H^2); value of 30 or more is indicative of obesity; value of less than 18.5 is indicative of undernutrition

Creatinine–height index (CHI) .. index or ratio sometimes used to assess body protein status

Diet history .... a detailed record of dietary intake obtainable from 24-hour recalls, food frequency questionnaires, food diaries, and similar methods

Gynoid obesity .... excess body fat that is placed predominantly within the hips and thighs

Kwashiorkor .... primarily a protein deficiency characterized by edema, growth failure, and muscle wasting

Malnutrition .... may mean any nutrition disorder but usually refers to long-term nutritional inadequacies or excesses

Marasmic kwashiorkor .... combination of chronic energy deficit and chronic or acute protein deficiency

Marasmus.................................. results from energy and protein deficiency, presenting with significant loss of body weight, skeletal muscle, and adipose tissue mass, but with serum protein concentrations relatively intact

Mid-arm muscle area (MAMA).. a more sensitive indicator of lean body mass than MAC or MAMC

Mid-upper arm circumference (MAC) .... an indicator of lean body mass and fat stores

Mid-upper arm muscle circumference (MAMC)............. an indicator of lean body mass calculated from the triceps skinfold thickness and the mid-upper arm circumference

Nitrogen balance .... condition in which nitrogen losses from the body are equal to nitrogen intake; the expected state of the healthy adult

Nutritional monitoring .... assessment of dietary or nutritional status at intermittent times with the aim of detecting changes in the dietary or nutritional status of a population

Nutrition screening .... a process used to identify individuals at nutrition risk or with nutritional problems

Obesity .... excessive accumulation of body fat; usually defined as 20% above desirable weight

Protein-calorie malnutrition (PCM) .... inadequate consumption of protein and energy, resulting in a gradual body wasting and increased susceptibility to infection

Recommended daily allowance (RDA) .... levels of intake of essential nutrients considered to be adequate to meet the nutritional needs of practically all healthy persons

Serum proteins .... proteins present in serum that are indicators of the body's visceral protein status (e.g., albumin, prealbumin, transferrin)

Skinfold thickness...................... double fold of skin and underlying subcutaneous tissue that is measured with skinfold calipers at various body sites

Waist-to-hip ratio (WHR) .... waist or abdominal circumference divided by the hip or gluteal circumference; method for assessing fat distribution

Study Guide

After completing the reading assignment, you should be able to answer the following questions in the spaces provided.

1. Define *nutritional status.*

2. Describe the unique nutritional needs for various developmental periods throughout the life cycle.

3. Describe the role cultural heritage and values may play in an individual's nutritional intake.

4. State 3 purposes of a nutritional assessment.

5. List and describe 5 factors that place an individual at nutritional risk.

6. Describe 4 sources of error that may occur when using the 24-hour diet recall.

7. Explain the clinical changes associated with each type of malnutrition:

   Obesity _____

   Marasmus _____

   Kwashiorkor _____

   Marasmus/kwashiorkor mix _____

REVIEW QUESTIONS

This test is for you and is intended to check your own mastery of the content. Answers are provided in Appendix A.

1. The balance between nutrient intake and nutrient requirements is described as:

   a) undernutrition.
   b) malnutrition.
   c) nutritional status.
   d) overnutrition.

2. To support the synthesis of maternal and fetal tissue during pregnancy, a weight gain of _____ pounds is recommended.

   a) 25 to 35 pounds
   b) 28 to 40 pounds
   c) 15 to 25 pounds
   d) Recommendation depends on BMI of mother at the start of the pregnancy.

3. Which of the following are normal, expected changes with aging?

   a) increase in energy needs
   b) increase in body water
   c) decrease in height
   d) increase in AP diameter of the chest

4. Which of the following data would be obtained as part of a nutritional screening?

   a) temperature, pulse, and respiration
   b) blood pressure and genogram
   c) weight and nutrition intake history
   d) serum creatinine levels

5. Current dietary guidelines recommend that complex carbohydrates comprise _____ % of total calorie intake.

   a) 30
   b) 40
   c) 60
   d) 75

6. The 24-hour recall of dietary intake:

   a) is an anthropometric measure of calories consumed.
   b) is a questionnaire or interview of everything eaten within the last 24 hours.
   c) is the same as a food frequency questionnaire.
   d) is a form of food diary.

7. The nutritional needs of a patient with trauma or major surgery:

   a) are met by fat reserves in obese individuals.
   b) may be two to three times greater than normal.
   c) can be met with intravenous fluids, supplemented with vitamins and electrolytes.
   d) are met by glycogen reserves.

8. Mary, a 15-year-old, has come for a school physical. During the interview, the examiner is told that menarche has not occurred. An explanation to be explored is:

   a) nutritional deficiency.
   b) alcohol intake.
   c) smoking history.
   d) possible elevated blood sugar.

9. Older adults are at risk for alteration in nutritional status. From the individuals described below, select the individual(s) who appear(s) *least at risk.*

   a) an 80-year-old widow who lives alone
   b) a 65-year-old widower who visits a senior center with a meal program 5 days a week
   c) a 70-year-old with poor dentition who lives with a son
   d) a 73-year-old couple with low income and no transportation

10. Body weight as a percentage of ideal body weight is calculated to assess for malnutrition. Severe malnutrition is diagnosed when current body weight is:

    a) 80% to 90% of ideal weight.
    b) 70% to 80% of ideal weight.
    c) less than 70% of ideal body weight.
    d) 120% of ideal body weight.

11. The examiner is completing an initial assessment for a patient being admitted to a long-term care facility. The patient is unable to stand for a measurement of height. In order to obtain this important anthropometric information the examiner may:

    a) measure the waist-to-hip circumference.
    b) estimate the body mass index.
    c) measure arm span.
    d) obtain a mid-upper arm muscle circumference to estimate skeletal muscle reserve.

12. A skin testing or anergy panel has been ordered for a patient. This test is done to:

    a) determine serum protein levels.
    b) determine the need for adult immunization.
    c) assess for excessive exposure to ultraviolet light.
    d) assess for immunocompetence.

SKILLS LABORATORY/CLINICAL SETTING

You are now ready for the clinical component of the nutritional assessment. The purpose of the clinical component is to practice the steps of the assessment on a peer in the skills laboratory and to achieve the following:

CLINICAL OBJECTIVES

1. Identify persons at risk for developing malnutrition.

2. Develop an appreciation for cultural influences on nutritional status.

3. Use anthropometric measures and laboratory data to assess the nutritional status of an individual.

4. Use nutritional assessment in the provision of health care.

5. Record the assessment findings accurately.

INSTRUCTIONS

Gather nutritional assessment forms and anthropometric equipment. Practice the steps of the *Admission Nutrition Screening Tool* on a peer in the skills laboratory. This will familiarize you with the appropriate history and give you practice computing the derived weight measures. Likely you will not have access to a peer's serum laboratory data; however, the history and physical exam data will give you all the data you need to make a clinical judgment on a well adult. Record your findings using one of the Assessment Forms that follow.

Next, practice the steps of the *Comprehensive Nutritional Assessment Form* on a peer in the skills laboratory or on a patient in the clinical setting. This will give you practice with a more detailed history, collecting food intake measures, physical examination signs, and performing anthropometric measures.

Finally, review the questions in the "Determine Your Nutritional Health" checklist with an aging adult. This is a three-step approach for nutrition screening of the elderly. The nutrition checklist is completed by the older person or caregiver and identifies major risk factors and indicators of poor nutritional status. Persons identified as being at risk should undergo Level 1 and/or Level 2 screening.

Level 1 screening is designed to identify individuals who may be candidates for preventive interventions such as home meal delivery, assistance with shopping or cooking, or nutrition education. The Level 1 screen collects data related to weight, height, eating habits, living environment, and functional status. The Level 2 screen identifies common nutritional disorders such as osteoporosis, protein-calorie malnutrition, and obesity. Data gathered for the Level 2 screen include a detailed history, physical examination, anthropometric measures, and laboratory tests.

NOTES

Admission Nutrition Screening Tool

A. DIAGNOSIS

If the patient has at least ONE of the following diagnoses, circle and proceed to section E to consider the patient
AT NUTRITIONAL RISK and stop here.

- Anorexia nervosa/bulimia nervosa
- Malabsorption (celiac sprue, ulcerative colitis, Crohn's disease, short bowel syndrome)
- Multiple trauma (closed-head injury, penetrating trauma, multiple fractures)
- Decubitus ulcers
- Major gastrointestinal surgery within the past year
- Cachexia (temporal wasting, muscle wasting, cancer, cardiac)
- Coma
- Diabetes
- End-stage liver disease
- End-stage renal disease
- Nonhealing wounds

B. NUTRITION INTAKE HISTORY

If the patient has at least ONE of the following symptoms, circle and proceed to section E to consider the patient
AT NUTRITIONAL RISK and stop here.

- Diarrhea (>500 mL $\times$ 2 days)
- Vomiting (>5 days)
- Reduced intake ($<1/2$ normal intake for >5 days)

C. IDEAL BODY WEIGHT STANDARDS

Compare the patient's current weight for height to the ideal body weight chart.
  If at $<80\%$ of ideal body weight, proceed to section E to consider the patient AT NUTRITIONAL RISK and stop here.

D. WEIGHT HISTORY

Any recent unplanned weight loss? No ___ Yes ___ Amount (lbs or kg) ___
  If yes, within the past ___ weeks or ___ months
  Current weight (lbs or kg) ___
  Usual weight (lbs of kg) ___
  Height (ft, in, or cm) ___

Find percentage of weight lost: $\dfrac{\text{usual wt} - \text{current wt}}{\text{usual wt}} \times 100 = $ _____ % wt loss

Compare the % wt loss with the chart values and circle appropriate value:

LENGTH OF TIME	SIGNIFICANT (%)	SEVERE (%)
1 week	1–2	>2
2–3 weeks	2–3	>3
1 months	4–5	>5
3 months	7–8	>8
5+ months	10	>10

If the patient has experienced a significant or severe weight loss, proceed to section E and consider the patient
AT NUTRITIONAL RISK.

E. NURSE ASSESSMENT

Using the above criteria, what is this patient's nutritional risk? (circle one)

  LOW NUTRITIONAL RISK

  AT NUTRITIONAL RISK

Nutrition Risk Classification: A Reproductive & Valid Tool for Nurses (Table 1—Admission Nutrition Screening Tool) by Debra S.
Kovacevich, et al. In *Nutrition in Clinical Practice* (February 1997) 12:20–25

Scored Patient-Generated Subjective Global Assessment (PG-SGA)

Patient ID Information

History (Boxes 1-4 are designed to be completed by the patient.)

1. Weight *(See Worksheet 1)*

In summary of my current and recent weight:

I currently weigh about _____ pounds
I am about _____ feet _____ tall

One month ago I weighed about _____ pounds
Six months ago I weighed about _____ pounds

During the past two weeks my weight has:

☐ decreased $_{(1)}$ ☐ not changed $_{(0)}$ ☐ increased $_{(0)}$

Box 1 [   ]

2. Food Intake: As compared to my normal intake, I would rate my food intake during the past month as:

☐ unchanged $_{(0)}$
☐ more than usual $_{(0)}$
☐ less than usual $_{(1)}$
  I am now taking:
    ☐ *normal food* but less than normal amount $_{(1)}$
    ☐ little solid food $_{(2)}$
    ☐ only liquids $_{(3)}$
    ☐ only nutritonal supplements $_{(3)}$
    ☐ very little of anything $_{(4)}$
    ☐ only tube feedings or only nutrition by vein $_{(0)}$

Box 2 [   ]

3. Symptoms: I have had the following problems that have kept me from eating enough during the past two weeks (check all that apply):

☐ no problems eating $_{(0)}$

☐ no appetite, just did not feel like eating $_{(3)}$

☐ nausea $_{(1)}$ ☐ vomiting $_{(3)}$
☐ constipation $_{(1)}$ ☐ diarrhea $_{(3)}$
☐ mouth sores $_{(2)}$ ☐ dry mouth $_{(1)}$
☐ things taste funny or have no taste $_{(1)}$ ☐ smells bother me $_{(1)}$
☐ problems swallowing $_{(2)}$ ☐ feel full quickly $_{(1)}$
☐ pain; where? $_{(3)}$_____
☐ other** $_{(1)}$ _____

   ** Examples: depression, money, or dental problems

Box 3 [   ]

4. Activities and Function: Over the past month, I would generally rate my activity as:

☐ normal with no limitations $_{(0)}$

☐ not my normal self, but able to be up and about with fairly normal activities $_{(1)}$

☐ not feeling up to most things, but in bed or chair less than half the day $_{(2)}$

☐ able to do little activity and spend most of the day in bed or chair $_{(3)}$

☐ pretty much bedridden, rarely out of bed $_{(3)}$

Box 4 [   ]

Additive Score of the Boxes 1-4 [   ] A

The remainder of this form will be completed by your doctor, nurse, or therapist. Thank you.

(Optional for completion by clinicians)

5. Disease and its relation to nutritional requirements *(See Worksheet 2)*

All relevant diagnoses (specify) _____

Primary disease stage (circle if known or appropriate)   I   II   III   IV   Other _____

Age _____

Numerical score from Worksheet 2 [   ] B

6. Metabolic Demand *(See Worksheet 3)*

Numerical score from Worksheet 3 [   ] C

7. Physical *(See Worksheet 4)*

Numerical score from Worksheet 4 [   ] D

Global Assessment *(See Worksheet 5)*

☐ Well-nourished or anabolic (SGA-A)
☐ Moderate or suspected malnutrition (SGA-B)
☐ Severely malnourished (SGA-C)

Total PG-SGA score

(Total numerical score of A+B+C+D above) [   ]
(See triage recommendations below)

Clinician Signature _____ RD RN PA MD DO Other ___   Date _____

Nutritional Triage Recommendations: Additive score is used to define specific nutritional interventions including patient & family education, symptom management including pharmacologic intervention, and appropriate nutrient intervention (food, nutritional supplements, enteral, or parenteral triage). First line nutrition intervention includes optimal symptom management.

0-1   No intervention required at this time. Re-assessment on routine and regular basis during treatment.
2-3   Patient & family education by dietitian, nurse, or other clinician with pharmacologic intervention as indicated by symptom survey (Box 3) and laboratory values as appropriate.
4-8   Requires intervention by dietitian, in conjunction with nurse or physician as indicated by symptoms survey (Box 3).
≥ 9   Indicates a critical need for improved symptom management and/or nutrient intervention options.

© FD Ottery, 2001   email: fdottery@btgc.com or noatpres1@aol.com

Worksheets for PG-SGA Scoring
© FD Ottery, 2001

Boxes 1-4 of the PG-SGA are designed to be completed by the patient. The PG-SGA numerical score is determined using 1) the parenthetical points noted in boxes 1-4 and 2) the worksheets below for items not marked with parenthetical points. Scores for boxes 1 and 3 are additive within each box and scores for boxes 2 and 4 are based on the highest scored item checked off by the patient.

Worksheet 1 - Scoring Weight (Wt) Loss

To determine score, use 1 month weight data if available. Use 6 month data only if there is no 1 month weight data. Use points below to score weight change and add one extra point if patient has lost weight during the past 2 weeks. Enter total point score in Box 1 of the PG-SGA.

Wt loss in 1 month	Points	Wt loss in 6 months
10% or greater	4	20% or greater
5-9.9%	3	10 -19.9%
3-4.9%	2	6 - 9.9%
2-2.9%	1	2 - 5.9%
0-1.9%	0	0 - 1.9%

Score for Worksheet 1 [   ]
Record in Box 1

Worksheet 2 - Scoring Criteria for Condition

Score is derived by adding 1 point for each of the conditions listed below that pertain to the patient.

Category	Points
Cancer	1
AIDS	1
Pulmonary or cardiac cachexia	1
Presence of decubitus, open wound, or fistula	1
Presence of trauma	1
Age greater than 65 years	1

Score for Worksheet 2 = [   ]
Record in Box B

Worksheet 3 - Scoring Metabolic Stress

Score for metabolic stress is determined by a number of variables known to increase protein & calorie needs. The score is additive so that a patient who has a fever of > 102 degrees (3 points) and is on 10 mg of prednisone chronically (2 points) would have an additive score for this section of 5 points.

Stress	none (0)	low (1)	moderate (2)	high (3)
Fever	no fever	>99 and <101	≥101 and <102	≥102
Fever duration	no fever	<72 hrs	72 hrs	> 72 hrs
Corticosteroids	no corticosteroids	low dose (<10mg prednisone equivalents/day)	moderate dose (≥10 and <30mg prednisone equivalents/day)	high dose steroids (≥30mg prednisone equivalents/day)

Score for Worksheet 3 = [   ]
Record in Box C

Worksheet 4 - Physical Examination

Physical exam includes a subjective evaluation of 3 aspects of body composition: fat, muscle, & fluid status. Since this is subjective, each aspect of the exam is rated for degree of deficit. Muscle deficit impacts point score more than fat deficit. Definition of categories: 0 = no deficit, 1+ = mild deficit, 2+ = moderate deficit, 3+ = severe deficit. Rating of deficit in these categories are *not* additive but are used to clinically assess the degree of deficit (or presence of excess fluid).

Fat Stores:

orbital fat pads	0	1+	2+	3+
triceps skin fold	0	1+	2+	3+
fat overlying lower ribs	0	1+	2+	3+
Global fat deficit rating	**0**	**1+**	**2+**	**3+**

Muscle Status:

temples (temporalis muscle)	0	1+	2+	3+
clavicles (pectoralis & deltoids)	0	1+	2+	3+
shoulders (deltoids)	0	1+	2+	3+
interosseous muscles	0	1+	2+	3+
scapula (latissimus dorsi, trapezius, deltoids)	0	1+	2+	3+
thigh (quadriceps)	0	1+	2+	3+
calf (gastrocnemius)	0	1+	2+	3+
Global muscle status rating	**0**	**1+**	**2+**	**3+**

Fluid Status:

ankle edema	0	1+	2+	3+
sacral edema	0	1+	2+	3+
ascites	0	1+	2+	3+
Global fluid status rating	**0**	**1+**	**2+**	**3+**

Point score for the physical exam is determined by the overall subjective rating of total body deficit.

No deficit	score = 0 points
Mild deficit	score = 1 point
Moderate deficit	score = 2 points
Severe deficit	score = 3 points

Score for Worksheet 4 = [   ]
Record in Box D

Worksheet 5 - PG-SGA Global Assessment Categories

Category	Stage A — Well-nourished	Stage B — Moderately malnourished or suspected malnutrition	Stage C — Severely malnourished
Weight	No wt loss OR Recent non-fluid wt gain	~5% wt loss within 1 month (or 10% in 6 months) OR No wt stabilization or wt gain (i.e., continued wt loss)	> 5% wt loss in 1 month (or >10% in 6 months) OR No wt stabilization or wt gain (i.e., continued wt loss)
Nutrient Intake	No deficit OR Significant recent improvement	Definite decrease in intake	Severe deficit in intake
Nutrition Impact Symptoms	None OR Significant recent improvement allowing adequate intake	Presence of nutrition impact symptoms (Box 3 of PG-SGA)	Presence of nutrition impact symptoms (Box 3 of PG-SGA)
Functioning	No deficit OR Significant recent improvement	Moderate functional deficit OR Recent deterioration	Severe functional deficit OR recent significant deterioration
Physical Exam	No deficit OR Chronic deficit but with recent clinical improvement	Evidence of mild to moderate loss of SQ fat &/or muscle mass &/or muscle tone on palpation	Obvious signs of malnutrition (e.g., severe loss of SQ tissues, possible edema)

Global PG-SGA rating (A, B, or C) = [   ]

NOTES

The warning signs of poor nutritional health are often overlooked. Use this checklist to find out if you or someone you know is at nutritional risk.

Read the statements below. Circle the number in the yes column for those that apply to you or someone you know. For each yes answer, score the number in the box. Total your nutritional score.

DETERMINE YOUR NUTRITIONAL HEALTH

	YES
I have an illness or condition that made me change the kind and/or amount of food I eat.	2
I eat fewer than 2 meals per day.	3
I eat few fruits or vegetables, or milk products.	2
I have 3 or more drinks of beer, liquor or wine almost every day.	2
I have tooth or mouth problems that make it hard for me to eat.	2
I don't always have enough money to buy the food I need.	4
I eat alone most of the time.	1
I take 3 or more different prescribed or over-the-counter drugs a day.	1
Without wanting to, I have lost or gained 10 pounds in the last 6 months.	2
I am not always physically able to shop, cook, and/or feed myself.	2
	TOTAL

Total Your Nutritional Score. If it's —

0-2 Good! Recheck your nutritional score in 6 months.

3-5 You are at moderate nutritional risk. See what can be done to improve your eating habits and lifestyle. Your office on aging, senior nutrition program, senior citizens center or health department can help. Recheck your nutritional score in 3 months.

6 or more You are at high nutritional risk. Bring this checklist the next time you see your doctor, dietitian, or other qualified health or social service professional. Talk with them about any problems you may have. Ask for help to improve your nutritional health.

These materials developed and distributed by the Nutrition Screening Initiative, a project of:

 AMERICAN ACADEMY OF FAMILY PHYSICIANS

 THE AMERICAN DIETETIC ASSOCIATION

 NATIONAL COUNCIL ON THE AGING, INC.

* **Remember that warning signs suggest risk but do not represent diagnosis of any condition.**

NOTES

Level 1 Screen

Body Weight

Measure height to the nearest inch and weight to the nearest pound. Record the values below and mark them on the Body Mass Index (BMI) scale to the right. Then use a straight edge (ruler) to connect the two points and circle the spot where this straight line crosses the center line (body mass index). Record the number below.

Healthy older adults should have a BMI between 24 and 27.

Height (in):_____
Weight (lbs):_____
Body Mass Index:_____
(number from center column)

Check any boxes that are true for the individual:

☐ Has lost or gained 10 pounds (or more) in the past 6 months.

☐ Body mass index <24

☐ Body mass index >27

For the remaining sections, please ask the individual which of the statements (if any) is true for him or her and place a check by each that applies.

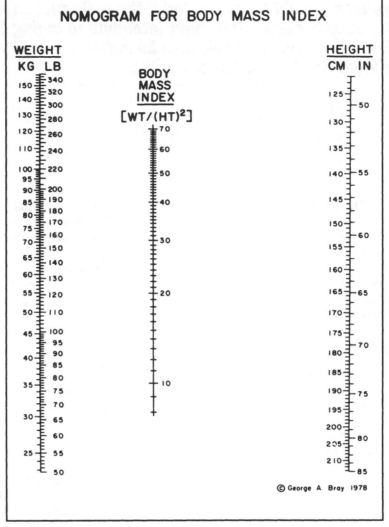

NOMOGRAM FOR BODY MASS INDEX

© George A. Bray 1978

Eating Habits

☐ Does not have enough food to eat each day

☐ Usually eats alone

☐ Does not eat anything on one or more days each month

☐ Has poor appetite

☐ Is on a special diet

☐ Eats vegetables two or fewer times daily

☐ Eats milk or milk products once or not at all daily

☐ Eats fruit or drinks fruit juice once or not at all daily

☐ Eats breads, cereals, pasta, rice, or other grains five or fewer times daily

☐ Has difficulty chewing or swallowing

☐ Has more than one alcoholic drink per day (if woman); more than two drinks per day (if man)

☐ Has pain in mouth, teeth, or gums

Reprinted with permission by the Nutrition Screening Initiative, a project of the American Academy of Family Physicians, the American Dietetic Association, and the National Council on the Aging, Inc., and funded in part by a grant from Ross Products Division, Abbott Laboratories.

Level 1 Screen *Continued*

A physician should be contacted if the individual has gained or lost 10 pounds unexpectedly or without intending to during the past 6 months. A physician should also be notified if the individual's body mass index is above 27 or below 22.

Living Environment

☐ Lives on an income of less than $6000 per year (per individual in the household)

☐ Lives alone

☐ Is housebound

☐ Is concerned about home security

☐ Lives in a home with inadequate heating or cooling

☐ Does not have a stove and/or refrigerator

☐ Is unable or prefers not to spend money on food (<$25-30 per person spent on food each week)

Functional Status

Usually or always needs assistance with (check each that apply):

☐ Bathing

☐ Dressing

☐ Grooming

☐ Toileting

☐ Eating

☐ Walking or moving about

☐ Traveling (outside the home)

☐ Preparing food

☐ Shopping for food or other necessities

If you have checked one or more statements on this screen, the individual you have interviewed may be at risk for poor nutritional status. Please refer this individual to the appropriate health care or social service professional in your area. For example, a dietitian should be contacted for problems with selecting, preparing, or eating a healthy diet, or a dentist if the individual experiences pain or difficulty when chewing or swallowing. Those individuals whose income, lifestyle, or functional status may endanger their nutritional and overall health should be referred to available community services: home-delivered meals, congregate meal programs, transportation services, counseling services (alcohol abuse, depression, bereavement, etc.), home health care agencies, day care programs, etc.

Please repeat this screen at least once each year – sooner if the individual has a major change in his or her health, income, immediate family (e.g., spouse dies), or functional status.

Reprinted with permission by the Nutrition Screening Initiative, a project of the American Academy of Family Physicians, the American Dietetic Association, and the National Council on the Aging, Inc., and funded in part by a grant from Ross Products Division, Abbott Laboratories.

Level 2 Screen

Complete the following screen by interviewing the patient directly and/or by referring to the patient chart. If you do not routinely perform all of the described tests or ask all of the listed questions, please consider including them, but do not be concerned if the entire screen is not completed. Please try to conduct a minimal screen on as many older patients as possible, and please try to collect serial measurements, which are extremely valuable in monitoring nutritional status. Please refer to the manual for additional information.

Anthropometrics

Measure height to the nearest inch and weight to the nearest pound. Record the values below and mark them on the Body Mass Index (BMI) scale to the right. Then use a straight edge (paper, ruler) to connect the two points and circle the spot where this straight line crosses the center line (body mass index). Record the number below; healthy older adults should have a BMI between 24 and 27; check the appropriate box to flag an abnormally high or low value.

NOMOGRAM FOR BODY MASS INDEX

BODY MASS INDEX [WT/(HT)^2]

© George A Bray 1978

Height (in):_____

Weight (lbs):_____

Body Mass Index
(weight/height^2):_____

Please place a check by any statement regarding BMI and recent weight loss that is true for the patient.

❑ Body mass index <24

❑ Body mass index >27

❑ Has lost or gained 10 pounds (or more) of body weight in the past 6 months

Record the measurement of mid-arm circumference to the nearest 0.1 centimeter and of triceps skinfold to the nearest 2 millimeters.

Mid-Arm Circumference (cm):_____
Triceps Skinfold (mm):_____
Mid-Arm Muscle Circumference (cm):_____

Refer to the table and check any abnormal values:

❑ Mid-arm muscle circumference <10th percentile

❑ Triceps skinfold <10th percentile

❑ Triceps skinfold >95th percentile

Note: mid-arm circumference (cm) - {0.314 x triceps skinfold (mm)}= mid-arm *muscle* circumference (cm)

For the remaining sections, please place a check by any statements that are true for the patient.

Laboratory Data

❑ Serum albumin below 3.5 g/dl

❑ Serum cholesterol below 160 mg/dl

❑ Serum cholesterol above 240 mg/dl

Drug Use

❑ Three or more prescription drugs, OTC medications, and/or vitamin/mineral supplements daily

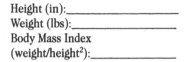

LEVEL 2 SCREEN Name: Date:

Reprinted with permission by the Nutrition Screening Initiative, a project of the American Academy of Family Physicians, the American Dietetic Association, and the National Council on the Aging, Inc., and funded in part by a grant from Ross Products Division, Abbott Laboratories.

Level 2 Screen *Continued*

Clinical Features

Presence of (check each that apply):

❑ Problems with mouth, teeth, or gums

❑ Difficulty chewing

❑ Difficulty swallowing

❑ Angular stomatitis

❑ Glossitis

❑ History of bone pain

❑ History of bone fractures

❑ Skin changes (dry, loose, nonspecific lesions, edema)

	Men		Women	
Percentile	55-65 y	65-75 y	55-65 y	65-75 y
Arm circumference (cm)				
10th	27.3	26.3	25.7	25.2
50th	31.7	30.7	30.3	29.9
95th	36.9	35.5	38.5	37.3
Arm muscle circumference (cm)				
10th	24.5	23.5	19.6	19.5
50th	27.8	26.8	22.5	22.5
95th	32.0	30.6	28.0	27.9
Triceps skinfold (mm)				
10th	6	6	16	14
50th	11	11	25	24
95th	22	22	38	36

From: Frisancho, A.R. New norms of upper limb fat and muscle areas for assessment of nutritional status. Am J Clin Nutr 1981; 34:2540-2545. © 1981 American Society for Clinical Nutrition.

Eating Habits

❑ Does not have enough food to eat each day

❑ Usually eats alone

❑ Does not eat anything on one or more days each month

❑ Has poor appetite

❑ Is on a special diet

❑ Eats vegetables two or fewer times daily

❑ Eats milk or milk products once or not at all daily

❑ Eats fruit or drinks fruit juice once or not at all daily

❑ Eats breads, cereals, pasta, rice, or other grains five or fewer times daily

❑ Has more than one alcoholic drink per day (if woman); more than two drinks per day (if man)

Living Environment

❑ Lives on an income of less than $6000 per year (per individual in the household)

❑ Lives alone

❑ Is housebound

❑ Is concerned about home security

❑ Lives in a home with inadequate heating or cooling

❑ Does not have a stove and/or refrigerator

❑ Is unable or prefers not to spend money on food (<$25-30 per person spent on food each week)

Functional Status

Usually or always needs assistance with (check each that apply):

❑ Bathing

❑ Dressing

❑ Grooming

❑ Toileting

❑ Eating

❑ Walking or moving about

❑ Traveling (outside the home)

❑ Preparing food

❑ Shopping for food or other necessities

Mental/Cognitive Status

❑ Clinical evidence of impairment, e.g., Folstein<26

❑ Clinical evidence of depressive illness, e.g., Beck Depression Inventory >15, Geriatric Depression Scale >5

Patients in whom you have identified one or more major indicator of poor nutritional status require immediate medical attention; if minor indicators are found, ensure that they are known to a health professional or to the patient's own physician. Patients who display risk factors of poor nutritional status should be referred to the appropriate health care or social service professional (dietitian, nurse, dentist, case manager, etc.).

UNIT 2

Approach to the Clinical Setting

Assessment Techniques and the Clinical Setting

PURPOSE

This chapter helps you to learn the assessment techniques of inspection, palpation, percussion, and auscultation; to learn the items of equipment needed for a complete physical examination; and to consider age-specific modifications you would make for the examination of individuals throughout the life cycle.

READING ASSIGNMENT

Jarvis, *Physical Examination and Health Assessment*, 4th ed., Chapter 9, pp. 161-174.

GLOSSARY

Study the following terms after completing the reading assignment. You should be able to cover the definition on the right and define the term out loud.

Amplitude .... (or intensity) how loud or soft a sound is

Duration .... the length of time a note lingers

Nosocomial infection .... an infection acquired during hospitalization

Ophthalmoscope .... an instrument that illuminates the internal eye structures, enabling the examiner to look through the pupil at the fundus (background) of the eye

Otoscope...................................... an instrument that illuminates the ear canal, enabling the examiner to look at the ear canal and tympanic membrane

Pitch... (or frequency) the number of vibrations (or cycles) per second of a note

Quality... (or timbre) a subjective difference in a sound due to the sound's distinctive overtones

Study Guide

After completing the reading assignment, you should be able to answer the following questions in the spaces provided.

1. Define and describe the technique of the 4 physical examination skills:

   Inspection _____

   Palpation _____

   Percussion _____

   Auscultation _____

2. Define the characteristics of the following percussion notes:

	Pitch	Amplitude	Quality	Duration
Resonance				
Hyperresonance				
Tympany				
Dull				
Flat				

3. Differentiate direct percussion from indirect percussion.

4. Relate the parts of the hands to palpation techniques used in assessment.

5. Differentiate between light, deep, and bimanual palpation.

6. List the two endpieces of the stethoscope and the conditions for which each is best suited.

7. Describe the environmental conditions to consider in preparing the examination setting.

8. List the 20 basic items of equipment necessary to conduct a complete physical examination on an adult.

9. Describe your own preparation as you encounter the patient for examination: your own dress, your demeanor, safety/universal precautions, sequence of examination steps, instructions to patient.

10. What age-specific considerations would you make for the examination of the:

Infant? _____

Toddler? _____

Preschooler? _____

School-aged child? _____

Adolescent? _____

Older adult? _____

Acutely ill person? _____

REVIEW QUESTIONS

This test is for you and is intended to check your own mastery of the content. Answers are provided in Appendix A.

1. Various parts of the hands are used during palpation. The part of the hand used for the assessment of vibration is (are) the:

   a) fingertips.
   b) index finger and thumb in opposition.
   c) dorsa of the hand.
   d) ulnar surface of the hand.

2. When performing indirect percussion, the stationary finger is struck:

   a) at the ulnar surface.
   b) at the middle joint.
   c) at the distal interphalangeal joint.
   d) wherever it is in contact with the skin.

3. The best description of the pitch of a sound wave obtained by percussion is:

   a) the intensity of the sound.
   b) the number of vibrations per second.
   c) the length of time the note lingers.
   d) the overtones of the note.

4. The bell of the stethoscope:

   a) is used for soft, low-pitched sounds.
   b) is used for high-pitched sounds.
   c) is held firmly against the skin.
   d) magnifies sound.

5. The ophthalmoscope has 5 apertures. Which aperture would be used to assess the eyes of a patient with undilated pupils?

   a) grid
   b) slit
   c) small
   d) large

6. At the conclusion of the examination, the examiner should:

   a) document findings before leaving the examining room.
   b) have findings confirmed by another practitioner.
   c) relate objective findings to the subjective findings for accuracy.
   d) summarize findings to the patient.

7. When the practitioner enters the examining room the infant patient is asleep. The practitioner would best start the exam with:

   a) height and weight.
   b) blood pressure.
   c) heart, lung, and abdomen.
   d) temperature.

8. The sequence of an examination changes from beginning with the thorax to that of head to toe with what age child?

   a) the infant
   b) the preschool child
   c) the school-aged child
   d) the adolescent

SKILLS LABORATORY/CLINICAL SETTING

Note that the clinical component of this chapter is combined with Chapter 10. Instructions and regional write-up forms are listed at the end of Chapter 10.

NOTES

General Survey, Measurement, Vital Signs

PURPOSE

This chapter helps you to learn the method of gathering data for a general survey on a patient and the techniques for measuring height, weight, and vital signs.

READING ASSIGNMENT

Jarvis, *Physical Examination and Health Assessment,* 4th ed., Chapter 10, pp. 175-206.

GLOSSARY

Study the following terms after completing the reading assignment. You should be able to cover the definition on the right and define the term out loud.

Auscultatory gap .... a brief time period when Korotkoff's sounds disappear during auscultation of blood pressure; common with hypertension

Bradycardia .... heart rate < 60 beats per minute in the adult

Sphygmomanometer .... instrument for measuring arterial blood pressure

Stroke volume .... amount of blood pumped out of the heart with each heartbeat

Tachycardia .... heart rate of > 100 beats per minute in the adult

STUDY GUIDE

After completing the reading assignment, you should be able to answer the following questions in the spaces provided.

1. List the significant information considered in each of the 4 areas of a general survey—physical appearance, body structure, mobility, and behavior.

2. Describe the normal posture and body build.

3. Note aspects of normal gait.

4. Describe the clinical appearance of the following variations in stature:

   Hypopituitary dwarfism _____

   Gigantism _____

   Acromegaly _____

   Achrondroplastic dwarfism _____

   Marfan's syndrome _____

   Endogenous obesity (Cushing's syndrome) _____

   Anorexia nervosa _____

5. State the normal weight range for a male 5'10" tall, medium frame _____; for a female 5' 4" tall, medium frame _____.

6. For serial weight measurements, what time of day would you instruct the person to have the weight measured? _____

7. Describe the technique for measuring head circumference and chest circumference on an infant.

8. What changes in height and in weight distribution would you expect for an adult in his or her 70s and 80s?

9. Describe the tympanic membrane thermometer, and compare its use to other forms of temperature measurement.

10. Describe 4 qualities to consider when assessing the pulse.

11. Relate the qualities of normal respirations to the appropriate approach to counting them.

12. Define and describe the relationships among the terms *blood pressure, systolic pressure, diastolic pressure, pulse pressure,* and *mean arterial pressure.*

13. List factors that affect blood pressure.

14. Relate the use of an improperly sized blood pressure cuff to the possible findings that may be obtained.

15. Explain the significance of Phase I, Phase IV, and Phase V Korotkoff's sounds during blood pressure measurement.

16. Given an apparently healthy 20-year-old adult, state the expected range for oral temperature, pulse, respirations, and blood pressure.

17. List the parameters of high normal blood pressure, Stage 1 or mild hypertension, and Stage 2 or moderate hypertension.

REVIEW QUESTIONS

This test is for you and is intended to check your own mastery of the content. Answers are provided in Appendix A.

1. The 4 areas to consider during the general survey are:

   a) ethnicity, sex, age, and socioeconomic status.
   b) physical appearance, sex, ethnicity, and affect.
   c) dress, affect, nonverbal behavior, and mobility.
   d) physical appearance, body structure, mobility, and behavior.

2. During the general survey part of the exam, gait is assessed. When walking, the base is usually:

   a) varied, depending upon the height of the person.
   b) equal to the length of the arm.
   c) as wide as the shoulder width.
   d) 1/2 of the height of the person.

3. A child, 18 months of age, is brought in for a health screening visit. To assess the height of the child:

   a) use a tape measure.
   b) use a horizontal measuring board.
   c) have the child stand on the upright scale.
   d) measure arm span to estimate height.

4. B. D. was delivered by cesarean section at 38 weeks of gestation because of fetal distress. She weighed 6 lb., 4 oz. This weight:

   a) is appropriate for gestational age.
   b) is small for gestational age.
   c) is large for gestational age.
   d) cannot be determined from available data.

5. During the 8th and 9th decades of life, physical changes occur. Height and weight:

   a) both increase.
   b) weight increases, height decreases.
   c) both decrease.
   d) both remain the same as during the 70s.

6. During an initial home visit, the patient's temperature is noted to be 97.4° F. This temperature:

   a) cannot be evaluated without a knowledge of the person's age.
   b) is below normal. The person should be assessed for possible hypothermia.
   c) should be retaken by the rectal route, since this best reflects core body temperature.
   d) should be reevaluated at the next visit before a decision is made.

7. Select the best description of an accurate assessment of a patient's pulse.

   a) Count for 15 seconds if pulse is regular.
   b) Begin counting with zero; count for 30 seconds.
   c) Count for 30 seconds and multiply by 2 for all cases.
   d) Count for 1 full minute; begin counting with zero.

8. After assessing the patient's pulse, the practitioner determines it to be "normal." This would be recorded as:

   a) 3+.
   b) 2+.
   c) 1+.
   d) 0.

9. Select the best description of an accurate assessment of a patient's respirations.

   a) Count for a full minute before taking the pulse.
   b) Count for 15 seconds and multiply by 4.
   c) Count after informing the patient where you are in the assessment process.
   d) Count for 30 seconds following pulse assessment.

10. Pulse pressure is:

    a) the difference between the systolic and diastolic pressure.
    b) a reflection of the viscosity of the blood.
    c) another way to express the systolic pressure.
    d) a measure of vasoconstriction.

11. The examiner is going to assess for coarctation of the aorta. In an individual with coarctation the thigh pressure would be:

    a) higher than in the arm.
    b) equal to that in the arm.
    c) there is no constant relationship. Findings are highly individual.
    d) lower than in the arm.

12. Mean arterial pressure is:

    a) the arithmetic average of systolic and diastolic pressures.
    b) the driving force of blood during systole.
    c) diastolic pressure plus one third pulse pressure.
    d) corresponding to Phase III Korotkoff's.

Skills Laboratory/Clinical Setting

You are now ready for the clinical component of Chapters 9 and 10. The purpose of the clinical component is to observe and describe the regional examination on a peer in the skills laboratory and to achieve the following.

Clinical Objectives

1. Observe and describe the significant characteristics of a general survey.

2. Measure height and weight and determine if findings are within normal range.

3. Gather vital signs data.

4. Record the physical examination findings accurately.

Instructions

Set up your section of the skills laboratory for a complete physical examination, attending to proper lighting, tables, and linen. Gather all equipment you will need for a complete physical examination, and make sure you are familiar with its mechanical operation. You will not use all the equipment today, but you will use it during the course of the semester, and this is the time to have it checked out.

Practice the steps of gathering data for a general survey, for height and weight, and vital signs on a peer. Record your findings using the regional write-up sheet that follows. The first section of the sheet is intended as a worksheet. It includes points for you to note that add up to the general survey. The bottom of the sheet has instructions for you to write the general survey statement; this is the topic sentence that will serve as an introduction for the complete physical examination write-up (see Jarvis, 4th ed., p. 200, for an example).

Notes

REGIONAL WRITE-UP—GENERAL SURVEY, VITAL SIGNS

Date _____

Patient _____ **Age** _____ **Sex** _____ **Occupation** _____

Examiner _____

Physical Examination

General Survey

1. Physical appearance
   Age _____
   Gender _____
   Level of consciousness _____
   Skin color _____
   Facial features _____

2. Body structure
   Stature _____
   Nutrition _____
   Symmetry _____
   Posture _____
   Position _____
   Body build, contour _____
   Any physical deformity _____

3. Mobility
   Gait _____
   Range of motion _____

4. Behavior
   Facial expression _____
   Mood and affect _____
   Speech _____
   Dress _____
   Personal hygiene _____

Measurement

1. Height _____ cm _____ ft/in
2. Weight _____ kg _____ lb

Vital Signs

1. Temperature _____
2. Pulse
   Rate _____
   Rhythm _____
3. Respirations _____
4. Blood pressure _____ R arm _____ L arm

Summary

(Write a summary of the general survey, including height, weight, and vital signs. This will serve as an introduction for the complete physical examination write-up.)

TABLE 10–1 Height and Weight Tables for Men and Women According to Frame, Ages 25–59

| HEIGHT* | | WEIGHT† | | |
Feet	Inches	Small Frame	Medium Frame	Large Frame
Men				
5	2	128–134	131–134	138–150
5	3	130–136	133–143	140–153
5	4	132–138	135–145	142–156
5	5	134–140	137–148	144–160
5	6	136–142	139–151	146–164
5	7	138–145	142–154	149–168
5	8	140–148	145–157	152–172
5	9	142–151	148–160	155–176
5	10	144–154	151–163	158–180
5	11	146–157	154–166	161–184
6	0	149–160	157–170	164–188
6	1	152–164	160–174	168–192
6	2	155–168	164–178	172–197
6	3	158–172	167–182	176–202
6	4	162–176	171–187	181–207
Women				
4	10	102–111	109–121	118–131
4	11	103–113	111–123	120–134
5	0	104–115	113–126	122–137
5	1	106–118	115–129	125–140
5	2	108–121	118–132	128–143
5	3	111–124	121–135	131–147
5	4	114–127	124–138	134–151
5	5	117–130	127–141	137–155
5	6	120–133	130–144	140–159
5	7	123–136	133–147	143–163
5	8	126–139	136–150	146–167
5	9	129–142	139–153	149–170
5	10	132–145	142–156	152–173
5	11	135–148	145–159	155–176
6	0	138–151	148–162	158–179

*Shoes with 1-inch heels.
†Weight in pounds. Men: allow 5 lb of clothing. Women: allow 3 lb of clothing.
Courtesy of Metropolitan Life Insurance Company, 1983.

Pain Assessment: The Fifth Vital Sign

PURPOSE

This chapter helps you to learn the structure and function of pain pathways, to understand the process of nociception, to understand the rationale and methods of pain assessment, and to accurately record the findings.

READING ASSIGNMENT

Jarvis, *Physical Examination and Health Assessment*, 4th ed., Chapter 11, pp. 207-220.

GLOSSARY

Study the following terms after completing the reading assignment. You should be able to cover the definition on the right and define the term out loud.

Cutaneous pain............................ pain originating from skin surface or subcutaneous structures

Modulation .... pain message is inhibited during this last phase of nociception

Neuropathic pain .... abnormal processing of pain message; burning, shooting in nature

Nociception................................. process whereby noxious stimuli are perceived as pain

Nociceptors .... specialized nerve endings that detect painful sensations

Pain... "An unpleasant sensory and emotional experience associated with actual or potential tissue damage, or described in terms of such damage. Pain is always subjective" (American Pain Society).

Perception .... conscious awareness of a painful sensation

Referred pain .... pain felt at a particular site, but originates from another location

Somatic pain .... originating from muscle, bone, joints, tendons, or blood vessels

Transduction .... first phase of nociception whereby the painful stimulus is changed into an action potential

Transmission .... second phase of nociception whereby the pain impulse moves from the spinal cord to the brain

Visceral pain .... originating from interior organs such as the gall bladder or stomach

STUDY GUIDE

After completing the reading assignment, you should be able to answer the following questions in the spaces provided.

1. Describe the process of nociception using the four phases of:

   Transduction

   Transmission

   Perception and

   Modulation

2. Identify the differences between nociceptive and neuropathic pain.

3. List various sources of pain.

4. Explain how acute and chronic pain differ in terms of nonverbal behaviors.

5. Identify the most reliable indicator of a person's pain.

6. Recall questions for an initial pain assessment.

7. Select pain assessment tools that are appropriate for adults, infants, and children.

8. Describe physical exam findings that may indicate pain.

9. Recall how poorly controlled acute and chronic pain adversely affect physiologic, social, and cognitive functioning.

CRITICAL THINKING QUESTIONS

1. What conditions are more likely to produce pain in the aging adult?

2. How would you modify your exam when the client reports having abdominal pain?

3. How would you assess for pain in an individual with dementia?

4. What would you say to someone who tells you that infants don't remember pain and that they are too little for the pain to have any damaging effect?

5. What would you say to a colleague who remarks that the individual with Alzheimer's disease does not feel pain and therefore does not require an analgesic?

Fill in the labels indicated on the following illustrations.

③ _____

② _____
The pain impulse moves from the spinal cord to the brain.

④ _____
Neurons from brain stem release neurotransmitters that block the pain impulse.

Neuron from brain stem

① _____
Noxious stimuli

① _____
• Injured tissue releases chemicals that propagate pain message.
• Action potential moves along an afferent fiber to the spinal cord.

Na+ K+
Na+ K+
Na+ Na+
       Na+
       Na+

PAT THOMAS

REVIEW QUESTIONS

This test is for you and is intended to check your own mastery of the content. The answers are provided in Appendix A.

1. At what phase during nociception does the individual become aware of a painful sensation?

   a) modulation
   b) transduction
   c) perception
   d) transmission

2. While taking a history, the patient describes a burning, painful sensation that moves around his toes and bottoms of his feet. These symptoms are suggestive of:

   a) nociceptive pain.
   b) neuropathic pain.

3. During your physical exam, your patient is diaphoretic, pale, and complains of pain directly over the LUQ of the abodomen. This would be categorized as:

   a) cutaneous pain.
   b) somatic pain.
   c) visceral pain.
   d) psychogenic pain.

4. While caring for the preterm infant, you are aware that:

   a) inhibitory neurotransmitters are in sufficient supply by 15 weeks' gestation.
   b) the fetus has less capacity to feel pain.
   c) repetitive blood draws have minimal long-term consequences.
   d) the preterm infant is more sensitive to painful stimuli.

5. The most reliable indicator of pain in the adult is:

   a) degree of physical functioning.
   b) nonverbal behaviors.
   c) MRI findings.
   d) the client's self report.

6. While examining a broken arm of a 4-year-old boy, select the appropriate assessment tool to evaluate his pain status.

   a) 0–10 numeric rating scale
   b) The Wong-Baker scale
   c) Simple descriptor scale
   d) 0–5 numeric rating scale

7. Normal age-related findings in the lower extremities of an 80-year-old woman would be:

   a) crepitus.
   b) joint swelling.
   c) diminished strength bilaterally.
   d) unilateral muscle atrophy.

8. When a person presents with acute pain of the abdomen, following the initial exam, it is best to withhold analgesia until diagnostic testing is completed and a diagnosis is made.

   a) True
   b) False

9. For elderly postoperative patients, poorly controlled acute pain places them at higher risk for:

   a) atelectasis.
   b) increased myocardial oxygen demand.
   c) impaired wound healing.
   d) all of the above.

10. A 30-year-old female reports having persistent intense pain in her right arm related to trauma sustained from a car accident 5 months ago. She states that the slightest touch or clothing can exacerbate the pain. This report is suggestive of:

a) referred pain.
b) psychogenic pain.
c) Complex Regional Pain I.
d) cutaneous pain.

11. The CRIES is an appropriate pain assessment tool for:

a) cognitively impaired elderly.
b) children ages 2–8 years.
c) infants.
d) preterm and term neonates.

12. A pain problem should be anticipated in a cognitively impaired older adult with a history of:

a) diabetes.
b) peripheral vascular disease.
c) COPD.
d) Parkinson's disease.

SKILLS LABORATORY/CLINICAL SETTING

You are now ready for the clinical component of the pain assessment. The purpose of the clinical component is to practice the examination on a peer in the skills laboratory or on a patient in the clinical setting and to achieve the following:

CLINICAL OBJECTIVES

1. Obtain an initial pain assessment on a classmate or patient.

2. Demonstrate a physical exam on painful area and identify abnormal findings.

3. Select appropriate pain assessment tools for further follow-up and monitoring.

4. Record the history and physical exam findings accurately, assess the nature of the pain, and develop an appropriate plan of care.

UNIT 3

Physical Examination

CHAPTER 12

Skin, Hair, and Nails

PURPOSE

This chapter helps you to learn the structure and function of the skin and its appendages; to understand the rationale for and the methods of inspection and palpation of the skin; and to record the assessment accurately.

READING ASSIGNMENT

Jarvis, *Physical Examination and Health Assessment*, 4th ed., Chapter 12, pp. 221-270.

AUDIO-VISUAL ASSIGNMENT

GLOSSARY

Study the following terms after completing the reading assignment. You should be able to cover the definition on the right and define the term out loud.

Alopecia .... (baldness) hair loss

Annular .... circular shape to skin lesion

Bulla .... elevated cavity containing free fluid larger than 1 cm diameter

Confluent .... skin lesions that run together

Crust .... thick, dried-out exudate left on skin when vesicles/pustules burst or dry up

Cyanosis .... dusky blue color to skin or mucous membranes due to increased amount of unoxygenated hemoglobin

Erosion .... scooped out, shallow depression in skin

Erythema .... intense redness of the skin due to excess blood in dilated superficial capillaries, as in fever or inflammation

Excoriation .... self-inflicted abrasion on skin due to scratching

Fissure .... linear crack in skin extending into dermis

Furuncle .... (boil) suppurative inflammatory skin lesion due to infected hair follicle

Hemangioma .... skin lesion due to benign proliferation of blood vessels in the dermis

Iris .... target shape of skin lesion

Jaundice .... yellow color to skin, palate, and sclera due to excess bilirubin in the blood

Keloid .... hypertrophic scar, elevated beyond site of original injury

Lichenification .... tightly packed set of papules that thickens skin, from prolonged intense scratching

Lipoma .... benign fatty tumor

Maceration .... softening of tissue by soaking

Macule .... flat skin lesion with only a color change

Nevus .... (mole) circumscribed skin lesion due to excess melanocytes

Nodule .... elevated skin lesion, > 1 cm diameter

Pallor .... excessively pale, whitish-pink color to lightly pigmented skin

Papule .... palpable skin lesion of < 1 cm diameter

Plaque .... skin lesion in which papules coalesce or come together

Pruritus .... itching

Purpura .... red-purple skin lesion due to blood in tissues from breaks in blood vessels

Pustule .... elevated cavity containing thick turbid fluid

Scale .... compact desiccated flakes of skin from shedding of dead skin cells

Telangiectasia .... skin lesion due to permanently enlarged and dilated blood vessels that are visible

Ulcer .... sloughing of necrotic inflammatory tissue that causes a deep depression in skin, extending into dermis

Vesicle .... elevated cavity containing free fluid up to 1 cm diameter

Wheal .... raised red skin lesion due to interstitial fluid

Zosteriform .... linear shape of skin lesion along a nerve route

STUDY GUIDE

After completing the reading assignment and the audio-visual assignment, you should be able to answer the following questions in the spaces provided.

1. List the 3 layers associated with the skin, and describe the contents of each layer.

2. Define 2 types of human hair.

3. Differentiate between sebaceous, eccrine, and apocrine glands.

4. List at least 5 functions of the skin.

5. List at least 6 variables that are external to the skin itself that can influence skin color.

6. Describe the appearance of pallor, erythema, cyanosis, and jaundice, both in light-skinned and in dark-skinned persons. State common causes of each.

7. List causes of changes in skin temperature, texture, moisture, mobility, and turgor.

8. Describe each grade on the 4-point grading scale for pitting edema.

9. Distinguish the terms *primary* versus *secondary* in reference to skin lesions.

10. The white linear markings that normally are visible through the nail and on the pink nail bed are termed _____.

11. Describe the following findings that are common variations on the infant's skin:

Mongolian spot _____

Café au lait spot _____

Erythema toxicum _____

Cutis marmorata _____

Physiologic jaundice _____

Milia _____

12. Describe the following findings that are common variations on the aging adult's skin:

Lentigines _____

Seborrheic keratosis _____

Actinic keratosis _____

Acrochordons (skin tags) _____

Sebaceous hyperplasia _____

13. Differentiate between these purpuric lesions: petechiae; ecchymosis; hematoma.

14. Differentiate between the appearance of the skin rash of these childhood illnesses: measles (rubeola); German measles (rubella); chicken pox (varicella).

15. List and describe 3 skin lesions associated with AIDS.

16. Contrast a furuncle with an abscess.

17. Describe the appearance of these conditions of the nails: koilonychia; paronychia; Beau's line; splinter hemorrhages; onycholysis; clubbing.

18. Define and give an example of the following primary skin lesions: macule; papule; plaque; nodule; tumor; wheal; vesicle; pustule.

And of these secondary lesions: crust; scale; fissure; erosion; ulcer; excoriation; scar; atrophic scar; lichenification; keloid.

Fill in the labels indicated on the following illustrations.

REVIEW QUESTIONS

This test is for you and is intended to check your own mastery of the content. Answers are provided in Appendix A.

1. Select the best description of the secretion of the eccrine glands.

   a) thick, milky
   b) dilute saline solution
   c) protective lipid substance
   d) keratin

2. Nevus is the medical term for:

   a) a freckle.
   b) a birthmark.
   c) an infected hair follicle.
   d) a mole.

3. To assess for early jaundice, you will assess:

   a) sclera and hard palate.
   b) nail beds.
   c) lips.
   d) all visible skin surfaces.

4. Checking for skin temperature is best accomplished by using:

   a) palmar surface of the hands.
   b) ventral surface of the hands.
   c) fingertips.
   d) dorsal surface of the hands.

5. Skin turgor is assessed by picking up a large fold of skin on the anterior chest under the clavicle. This is done to determine the presence of:

   a) edema.
   b) dehydration.
   c) vitiligo.
   d) scleroderma.

6. You note a lesion during an examination. Select the description that is most complete.

   a) raised, irregular lesion, the size of a quarter, located on dorsum of left hand
   b) open lesion with no drainage or odor approximately 1/4 inch in diameter
   c) pedunculated lesion below left scapula with consistent red color, no drainage or odor
   d) dark brown, raised lesion, with irregular border, on dorsum of right foot, 3 cm in size with no drainage

7. You examine nail beds for clubbing. The normal angle between the nail base and the nails is:

   a) 60 degrees.
   b) 100 degrees.
   c) 160 degrees.
   d) 180 degrees.

8. The capillary beds should refill after being depressed in:

   a) < 1 second.
   b) > 2 seconds.
   c) 1–2 seconds.
   d) time is not significant as long as color returns.

9. During a routine visit, M. B., aged 78, asks about small, round, flat, brown macules on the hands. Your best response after examining the areas is:

   a) "These are the result of sun exposure and do not require treatment."
   b) "These are related to exposure to the sun. They may become cancerous."
   c) "These are the skin tags that occur with aging. No treatment is required."
   d) "I'm glad you brought this to my attention. I will arrange for a biopsy."

10. An area of thin, shiny skin with decreased visibility of normal skin markings is called:

    a) lichenification.
    b) plaque.
    c) atrophy.
    d) keloid.

11. Flattening of the angle between the nail and its base is:

    a) found in subacute bacterial endocarditis.
    b) a description of spoon-shaped nails.
    c) related to calcium deficiency.
    d) described as clubbing.

12. The configuration for individual lesions arranged in circles or arcs, as occurs with ringworm, is called:

    a) linear.
    b) clustered.
    c) annular.
    d) gyrate.

13. The "A" in the ABCDE rule stands for:

    a) accuracy.
    b) appearance.
    c) asymmetry.
    d) attenuated.

14. A risk factor for melanoma is:

    a) brown eyes.
    b) darkly pigmented skin.
    c) skin that freckles or burns before tanning.
    d) use of sunscreen products.

15. Lyme disease is more prevalent:

    a) in May through September.
    b) along the West Coast.
    c) in children under age 3.
    d) in those participating in water sports.

16. Cutaneous anthrax:

    a) incubation is 10–15 days.
    b) is completely curable with antibiotic treatment.
    c) has absence of pain or edema.
    d) forms pustular, umbilicated lesions.

Match column A to column B—items in column B may be used more than once.

Column A—descriptor   **Column B—skin layer**

17. ___ basal cell layer   a) epidermis

18. ___ aids protection by cushioning b) dermis

19. ___ collagen   c) subcutaneous layer

20. ___ adipose tissue

21. ___ uniformly thin

22. ___ stratum corneum

23. ___ elastic tissue

Column A—descriptor

24. ___ pallor

25. ___ erythema

26. ___ cyanosis

27. ___ jaundice

Column B—color change

a) intense redness of the skin due to excess blood in the dilated superficial capillaries

b) bluish mottled color that signifies decreased perfusion

c) absence of red-pink tones from the oxygenated hemoglobin in blood

d) increase in bilirubin in the blood causing a yellow color in the skin

Column A—descriptor

28. ___ tiny, punctate red macules and papules on the cheeks, trunk, chest, back, and buttocks

29. ___ lower half of body turns red, upper half blanches

30. ___ transient mottling on trunk and extremities

31. ___ bluish color around the lips, hands, and fingernails, pigmentation, and feet and toenails

32. ___ large round or oval patch of light brown usually present at birth

33. ___ yellowing of skin, sclera, and mucous membranes due to increased numbers of red blood cells hemolyzed following birth

34. ___ yellow-orange color in light-skinned persons from large amounts of foods containing carotene

Column B—skin color change

a) harlequin

b) erythema toxicum

c) acrocyanosis

d) physiologic jaundice

e) carotenemia

f) café au lait

g) cutis marmorata

SKILLS LABORATORY/CLINICAL SETTING

You are now ready for the clinical component of the integumentary system. Usually the clinical examination of the integumentary system is performed along with the examination of each particular body region. The purpose of practicing the steps of this examination separately is so that you begin to think of the skin and its appendages as a separate organ system, and so that you learn the components of skin examination.

CLINICAL OBJECTIVES

1. Inspect and palpate the skin, noting its color, vascularity, edema, moisture, temperature, texture, thickness, mobility and turgor, and any lesions.

2. Inspect the fingernails, noting color, shape, and any lesions.

3. Inspect the hair, noting texture, distribution, and any lesions.

4. Record the history and physical examination findings accurately, reach an assessment of the health state, and develop a plan of care.

Instructions

Prepare the examination setting. Wash your hands. Practice the steps of the exam on a peer in the skills laboratory, giving appropriate instructions as you proceed. Choosing a peer from an ethnic background other than your own will further heighten your recognition of the range of normal skin tones. Record your findings using the regional write-up sheet that follows. The front of the page is intended as a worksheet; the back of the page is intended for your narrative summary recording using the SOAP format.

Note the student performance checklist that follows the regional write-up sheet. It lists the essential behaviors you should display as an examiner, and it may be used by your clinical instructor to evaluate your clinical teaching of the skin self-examination.

Notes

REGIONAL WRITE-UP—SKIN, HAIR, AND NAILS

Date_____

Patient _____ Age ___ Sex ___ Occupation _____

Examiner _____

I. Health History

	No	Yes, explain
1. Any previous **skin disease**?		
2. Any change in skin color or **pigmentation**?		
3. Any changes in a **mole**?		
4. Excessive **dryness** or **moisture**?		
5. Any skin **itching**?		
6. Any excess **bruising**?		
7. Any skin **rash** or **lesions**?		
8. Taking any **medications**?		
9. Any recent hair loss?		
10. Any change in nails?		
11. Any environmental hazards for skin?		
12. How do you take care of skin?		

II. Physical Examination

A. Inspect and palpate skin:

Color _____

Pigmentation _____

Temperature _____

Moisture _____

Texture _____

Thickness _____

Any edema _____

Mobility and turgor _____

Vascularity and bruising _____

Any lesions _____

B. Inspect and palpate hair:

Color _____

Texture _____

Distribution _____

Any lesions _____

C. Inspect and palpate nails:

Shape and contour _____

Consistency _____

Distribution _____

Color _____

D. Teach skin self-examination

REGIONAL WRITE-UP—SKIN, HAIR, AND NAILS

Summarize your findings using the SOAP format.

Subjective (Reason for seeking care, health history)

Objective (Physical exam findings)

Record distribution of rash or lesions below

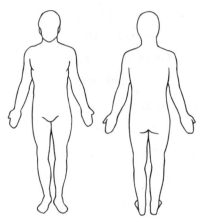

Assessment (Assessment of problem, diagnosis)

Plan (Diagnostic evaluation, follow-up care, teaching)

STUDENT PERFORMANCE CHECKLIST

TEACHING SKIN SELF-EXAMINATION (SSE)

	S	U	Comments
I. Cognitive			
1. Explain:			
a. Why skin is examined			
b. Who should perform skin self-examination			
c. Frequency of skin exam			
2. Define the ABCDE rule			
3. Describe any equipment the patient may need			
II. Performance			
1. Explains to patient need for SSE			
2. Instructs patient on technique of SSE by:			
a. demonstrating the order and body positioning for inspecting skin			
b. describing normal skin characteristics			
c. describing abnormal findings to look for			
3. Instructs patient to report unusual findings to nurse or physician at once			

CHAPTER 13

Head and Neck, Including Regional Lymphatics

PURPOSE

This chapter helps you to learn the location and function of structures in the head and neck; to learn to perform inspection and palpation of the head and neck; and to record the assessment accurately.

READING ASSIGNMENT

Jarvis, *Physical Examination and Health Assessment,* 4th ed., Chapter 13 pp. 271-296.

AUDIO-VISUAL ASSIGNMENT

Jarvis, *Saunders Physical Examination Video Assessment Series: Head, Eyes, and Ears*

GLOSSARY

Study the following terms after completing the reading assignment. You should be able to cover the definition on the right and define the term out loud.

Bruit.. blowing, swooshing sound heard through the stethoscope over an area of abnormal blood flow

Goiter.. increase in size of thyroid gland that occurs with hyperthyroidism

Lymphadenopathy.................... enlargement of the lymph nodes due to infection, allergy, or neoplasm

Macrocephalic.......................... abnormally large head

Microcephalic........................... abnormally small head

Normocephalic........................... round symmetric skull that is appropriately related to body size

Torticollis................................. head tilt due to shortening or spasm of one sternomastoid muscle

STUDY GUIDE

After completing the reading assignment and the audio-visual assignment, you should be able to answer the following questions in the spaces provided.

1. The major neck muscles are the _____ and

   _____.

2. Name the borders of two regions in the neck, the anterior triangle, and the posterior triangle.

3. List the facial structures that should appear symmetric when inspecting the head.

4. Describe the characteristics of lymph nodes often associated with:

   Acute infection

   Chronic inflammation

   Cancer

5. Differentiate *caput succedaneum* from *cephalhematoma* in the newborn infant.

6. Describe the tonic neck reflex in the infant.

7. Describe the characteristics of normal cervical lymph nodes during childhood.

8. List the condition(s) associated with parotid gland enlargement.

9. Describe the facial characteristics that occur with Down's syndrome.

10. Contrast the facial characteristics of hyperthyroidism versus hypothyroidism.

ASSESSMENT VIDEO CRITICAL THINKING QUESTIONS

Discussion answers to these questions are in the Instructor's Manual for *Physical Examination and Health Assessment*, 4th ed.

1. How do examination techniques and findings differ when palpating the head of an adult and the head of an infant?

2. Describe characteristics of normal and abnormal cervical lymph nodes.

Fill in the labels indicated on the following illustrations.

REVIEW QUESTIONS

This test is for you and is intended to check your own mastery of the content. Answers are provided in Appendix A.

1. Identify the facial bone that articulates at a joint instead of a suture.

   a) zygomatic
   b) maxilla
   c) nasal
   d) mandible

2. Identify the blood vessel that runs diagonally across the sternomastoid muscle.

   a) temporal artery
   b) carotid artery
   c) external jugular vein
   d) internal jugular vein

3. The isthmus of the thyroid gland lies just below the:

   a) mandible.
   b) cricoid cartilage.
   c) hyoid cartilage.
   d) thyroid cartilage.

4. Select the statement that is true regarding cluster headaches.

   a) May be precipitated by alcohol and daytime napping.
   b) Usual occurrence is two per month, each lasting 1 to 3 days.
   c) Characterized as throbbing.
   d) Tend to be supraorbital, retro-orbital or frontotemporal.

5. Select the symptom that is least likely to indicate a possible malignancy.

   a) history of radiation therapy to head, neck, or upper chest
   b) history of using chewing tobacco
   c) history of large alcohol consumption
   d) tenderness

6. Providing resistance while the patient shrugs the shoulders is a test of the status of cranial nerve:

   a) II
   b) V
   c) IX
   d) XI

7. Upon examination, the fontanels should feel:

   a) tense or bulging.
   b) depressed or sunken.
   c) firm, slightly concave, and well defined.
   d) pulsating.

8. If the thyroid gland is enlarged bilaterally, which of the following maneuvers is appropriate?

   a) Check for deviation of the trachea.
   b) Listen for a bruit over the carotid arteries.
   c) Listen for a murmur over the aortic area.
   d) Listen for a bruit over the thyroid lobes.

9. It is normal to palpate a few lymph nodes in the neck of a healthy person. What are the characteristics of these nodes?

   a) mobile, soft, nontender
   b) large, clumped, tender
   c) matted, fixed, tender, hard
   d) matted, fixed, nontender

10. Cephalhematoma is associated with:

   a) subperiosteal hemorrhage.
   b) craniotabes.
   c) bossing.
   d) congenital syphilis.

11. Normal cervical lymph nodes are:

   a) smaller than 1 cm.
   b) warm to palpation.
   c) fixed.
   d) firm.

12. A throbbing, unilateral pain associated with nausea, vomiting, and photophobia is characteristic of:

   a) cluster headache.
   b) subarachnoid hemorrhage.
   c) migraine headache.
   d) tension headache.

Match column A with column B.

Column A—lymph nodes

13. _____ Preauricular
14. _____ Posterior auricular
15. _____ Occipital
16. _____ Submental
17. _____ Submandibular
18. _____ Jugulodigastric
19. _____ Superficial cervical
20. _____ Deep cervical
21. _____ Posterior cervical
22. _____ Supraclavicular

Column B—location

a) above and behind the clavicle
b) deep under the sternomastoid muscle
c) in front of the ear
d) in the posterior triangle along the edge of the trapezius muscle
e) superficial to the mastoid process
f) at the base of the skull
g) halfway between the angle and the tip of the mandible
h) behind the tip of the mandible
i) under the angle of the mandible
j) overlying the sternomastoid muscle

SKILLS LABORATORY/CLINICAL SETTINGS

You are now ready for the clinical component of the head and neck chapter. The purpose of the clinical component is to practice the steps of the head and neck examination on a peer in the skills laboratory and to achieve the following objectives.

CLINICAL OBJECTIVES

1. Collect a health history related to pertinent signs and symptoms of the head and neck.

2. Inspect and palpate the skull noting size, contour, lumps, or tenderness.

3. Inspect the face noting facial expression, symmetry, skin characteristics, lesions.

4. Inspect and palpate the neck for symmetry, range of motion, and integrity of lymph nodes, trachea, and thyroid gland.

5. Record the findings systematically, reach an assessment of the health state, and develop a plan of care.

INSTRUCTIONS

Prepare the examination setting. Wash your hands. Practice the steps of the exam on a peer in the skills laboratory, giving appropriate instructions as you proceed. Record your findings using the regional write-up sheet that follows. The front of the page is intended as a worksheet; the back of the page is intended for your narrative summary recording using the SOAP format.

NOTES

REGIONAL WRITE-UP—HEAD AND NECK

Date_____

Patient _____ Age ____ Sex ___ Occupation_____

Examiner _____

I. Health History

	No	Yes, explain
1. Any unusually frequent or unusually severe **headaches**?		
2. Any **head injury**?		
3. Experienced any **dizziness?**		
4. Any neck **pain**?		
5. Any **lumps** or **swelling** in head or neck?		
6. Any surgery on head or neck?		

II. Physical Examination

A. Inspect and palpate the skull

General size and contour _____

Deformities, lumps, tenderness _____

Temporal artery _____

Temporomandibular joint _____

B. Inspect the face

Facial expression _____

Symmetry of structures _____

Involuntary movements _____

Edema _____

Masses or lesions _____

Color and texture of skin _____

C. Inspect the neck

Symmetry _____

Range of motion, active _____

Test strength of cervical muscles _____

Abnormal pulsations _____

Enlargement of thyroid _____

Enlargement of lymph and salivary glands _____

D. Palpate the lymph nodes

Exact location _____

Size and shape _____

Presence or absence of tenderness _____

Freely movable, adherent to deeper structures, or matted together _____

Presence of surrounding inflammation _____

Texture (hard, soft, firm) _____

E. Palpate the trachea

F. Palpate the thyroid gland

G. Auscultate the thyroid gland (if enlarged)

REGIONAL WRITE-UP—HEAD AND NECK

Summarize your findings using the SOAP format.

Subjective (Reason for seeking care, health history)

Objective (Physical exam findings)

Assessment (Assessment of health state or problem, diagnosis)

Plan (Diagnostic evaluation, follow-up care, patient teaching)

CHAPTER 14

Eyes

PURPOSE

This chapter helps you to learn the structure and function of the external and internal components of the eyes; to learn the methods of examination of vision, external eye, and ocular fundus; and to record the assessment accurately.

READING ASSIGNMENT

Jarvis, *Physical Examination and Health Assessment,* 4th ed., Chapter 14, pp. 297-340.

AUDIO-VISUAL ASSIGNMENT

Jarvis, *Saunders Video Assessment Series: Head, Eyes, and Ears*

GLOSSARY

Study the following terms after completing the reading assignment. You should be able to cover the definition on the right and define the term out loud.

Accommodation .... adaptation of the eye for near vision by increasing the curvature of the lens

Anisocoria .... unequal pupil size

Arcus senilis .... gray-white arc or circle around the limbus of the iris that is common with aging

Argyll Robertson pupil .... pupil does not react to light; does constrict with accommodation

Astigmatism .... refractive error of vision due to differences in curvature in refractive surfaces of the eye (cornea and lens)

A-V crossing .... crossing paths of an artery and vein in the ocular fundus

Bitemporal hemianopsia .... loss of both temporal visual fields

Blepharitis .... inflammation of the glands and eyelash follicles along the margin of the eyelids

Cataract .... opacity of the lens of the eye that develops slowly with aging and gradually obstructs vision

Chalazion .... infection or retention cyst of a meibomian gland, showing as a beady nodule on the eyelid

Conjunctivitis .... infection of the conjunctiva, "pinkeye"

Cotton-wool area .... abnormal soft exudates visible as gray-white areas on the ocular fundus

Cup-disc ratio .... ratio of the width of the physiologic cup to the width of the optic disc, normally 1/2 or less

Diopter .... unit of strength of the lens settings on the ophthalmoscope that changes focus on the eye structures

Diplopia .... double vision

Drusen .... benign deposits on the ocular fundus that show as round yellow dots and occur commonly with aging

Ectropion .... lower eyelid loose and rolling outward

Entropion .... lower eyelid rolling inward

Exopthalmos .... protruding eyeballs

Fovea .... area of keenest vision at the center of the macula on the ocular fundus

Glaucoma .... a group of eye diseases characterized by increased intraocular pressure

Hordeolum .... (stye) red, painful pustule that is a localized infection of hair follicle at eyelid margin

Lid lag .... the abnormal white rim of sclera visible between the upper eyelid and the iris when a person moves the eyes downward

Macula .... round darker area of the ocular fundus that mediates vision only from the central visual field

Microaneurysm .... abnormal finding of round red dots on the ocular fundus that are localized dilatations of small vessels

Miosis .... constricted pupils

Mydriasis .... dilated pupils

Myopia .... "nearsighted"; refractive error in which near vision is better than far vision

Nystagmus .... involuntary, rapid, rhythmic movement of the eyeball

OD .... oculus dexter, or right eye

Optic atrophy .... pallor of the optic disc due to partial or complete death of optic nerve

Optic disc .... area of ocular fundus in which blood vessels exit and enter

OS .... oculus sinister, or left eye

Papilledema .... stasis of blood flow out of the ocular fundus; sign of increased intracranial pressure

Presbyopia .... decrease in power of accomodation that occurs with aging

Pterygium .... triangular opaque tissue on the nasal side of the conjunctiva that grows toward the center of the cornea

Ptosis .... drooping of upper eyelid over the iris and possibly covering pupil

Red reflex .... red glow that appears to fill the person's pupil when first visualized through the ophthalmoscope

Strabismus .... (squint, crossed eye) disparity of the eye axes

Xanthelasma .... soft, raised yellow plaques occurring on the skin at the inner corners of the eyes

STUDY GUIDE

After completing the reading assignment and the audio-visual assignment, you should be able to answer the following questions in the spaces provided.

1. Name the 6 sets of extraocular muscles and the cranial nerve that innervates each one.

2. Name the 3 concentric coats of the eyeball.

3. Name the functions of the ciliary body, the pupil, and the iris.

4. Describe the compartments of the eye.

5. Describe how an image formed on the retina compares with its actual appearance in the outside world.

6. Describe the lacrimal system.

7. Define pupillary light reflex, fixation, and accommodation.

8. Concerning the pupillary light reflex, describe and contrast a direct light reflex with a consensual light reflex.

9. Identify common age-related changes in the eye.

10. Discuss the most common causes of decreased visual function in the older adult.

11. Explain the statement that normal visual acuity is 20/20.

12. Describe the method of testing for presbyopia.

13. To test for accommodation, the person focuses on a distant object, then shifts the gaze to a near object about 6 inches away. At near distance, you would expect the pupils to _____ (dilate/con-strict), and the axes of the eyes to _____.

14. Concerning malalignment of the eye axes, contrast phoria with tropia.

15. Describe abnormal findings of tissue color that are possible on the conjunctiva and sclera, and their significance.

16. Describe the method of everting the upper eyelid for examination.

17. Contrast *pinguecula* with *pterygium.*

18. Contrast the use of the negative diopter or red lens settings with the positive diopter or black lens settings on the ophthalmoscope.

19. Contrast a *scleral crescent* with a *pigment crescent*.

20. Explain the rationale for testing for strabismus during early childhood.

21. Describe these findings and explain their significance: epicanthal fold; pseudostrabismus; Mongolian slant; ophthalmia neonatorum; Brushfield's spots.

22. Describe the following 4 types of "red eye" and explain their significance: conjunctivitis; subconjunctival hemorrhage; iritis; acute glaucoma.

ASSESSMENT VIDEO CRITICAL THINKING QUESTIONS

Discussion answers to these questions are in the Instructor's Manual for *Physical Examination and Health Assessment*, 4th ed.

1. What additional vision tests could you use, and why would you use them?

2. Describe the following abnormal findings, which may be found during inspection of the eyelids: exophthalmos, ptosis, ectropion, hordeolum, chalazion, and carcinoma.

Fill in the labels indicated on the following illustrations.

REVIEW QUESTIONS

This test is for you and is intended to check your own mastery of the content. Answers are provided in Appendix A.

1. The palpebral fissure is:

    a) the border between the cornea and sclera.
    b) the open space between the eyelids.
    c) the angle where the eyelids meet.
    d) visible on the upper and lower lids at the inner canthus.

2. The corneal reflex is mediated by cranial nerves:

    a) II and III.
    b) II and VI.
    c) V and VII.
    d) VI and IV.

3. The retinal structures viewed through the ophthalmoscope are:

    a) the optic disc, the retinal vessels, the general background, and the macula.
    b) the cornea, the lens, the choroid, and the ciliary body.
    c) the optic papilla, the sclera, the retina, and the iris.
    d) the pupil, the sclera, the ciliary body, and the macula.

4. The examiner records "positive consensual light reflex." This is:

    a) the convergence of the axes of the eyeballs.
    b) the simultaneous constriction of the other pupil when one eye is exposed to bright light.
    c) a reflex direction of the eye toward an object attracting a person's attention.
    d) the adaptation of the eye for near vision.

5. Several changes occur in the eye with the aging process. The thickening and yellowing of the lens is referred to as:

    a) presbyopia.
    b) floaters.
    c) macular degeneration.
    d) senile cataract.

6. Be alert to symptoms that may constitute an eye emergency. Identify the symptom(s) that should be referred immediately.

    a) floaters
    b) epiphora
    c) sudden onset of vision change
    d) photophobia

7. Visual acuity is assessed with:

    a) the Snellen eye chart.
    b) an ophthalmoscope.
    c) the Hirschberg test.
    d) the confrontation test.

8. The cover test is used to assess for:

    a) nystagmus.
    b) peripheral vision.
    c) muscle weakness.
    d) visual acuity.

9. When using the ophthalmoscope, you would:

    a) remove your own glasses and approach the patient's left eye with your left eye.
    b) leave light on in the examining room and remove glasses from the patient.
    c) remove glasses and set the diopter setting at 0.
    d) use the smaller white light and instruct the patient to focus on the ophthalmoscope.

10. The six muscles that control eye movement are innervated by cranial nerves:

    a) II, III, V.
    b) IV, VI, VII.
    c) III, IV, VI.
    d) II, III, VI.

11. Conjunctivitis is always associated with:

    a) absent red reflex.
    b) reddened conjunctiva.
    c) impairment of vision.
    d) fever.

12. A patient has blurred peripheral vision. You suspect glaucoma, and test the visual fields. A person with normal vision would see your moving finger temporally at:

a) 50 degrees.
b) 60 degrees.
c) 90 degrees.
d) 180 degrees.

13. A person is known to be blind in the left eye. What happens to the pupils when the right eye is illuminated by a penlight beam?

a) No response in both.
b) Both pupils constrict.
c) Right pupil constricts, left has no response.
d) Left pupil constricts, right has no response.

14. Use of the ophthalmoscope: an interruption of the red reflex occurs when:

a) there is an opacity in the cornea or lens.
b) the patient has pathology of the optic tract.
c) the blood vessels are tortuous.
d) the pupils are constricted.

15. One cause of visual impairment in aging adults is:

a) strabismus.
b) glaucoma.
c) amblyopia.
d) retinoblastoma.

16. Briefly describe the method of assessing the six cardinal fields of vision.

SKLLS LABORATORY/CLINICAL SETTING

You are now ready for the clinical component of the eye examination. The purpose of the clinical component is to practice the steps of the examination on a peer in the skills laboratory. Note that the first practice session usually takes a long time because there are so many separate steps. Be aware that success with the use of the ophthalmoscope is hard to achieve during the first practice session. Make sure you are holding the instrument correctly and practice focusing on various objects about the room before you try to look at a person's fundus. When you do examine a peer's eye, make sure to offer occasional rest times. It is very tiring for the "patient" to have the ophthalmoscope light shining in the eye. During the first practice session, aim for finding the red reflex and a retinal vessel or two; if you can locate the optic disc, so much the better.

CLINICAL OBJECTIVES

1. Collect a health history related to pertinent signs and symptoms of the eye system.

2. Demonstrate and explain assessment of visual acuity, visual fields, external eye structures, and ocular fundus.

3. Record the history and physical examination findings accurately, reach an assessment of the health state, and develop a plan of care.

INSTRUCTIONS

Prepare the examination setting. Wash your hands. Practice the steps of the exam on a peer in the skills laboratory, giving appropriate instructions as you proceed. Record your findings using the regional writeup sheet that follows. The front of the page is intended as a worksheet; the back of the page is intended for your narrative summary recording using the SOAP format.

REGIONAL WRITE-UP—EYES

Date _____

Patient _____ Age _____ Sex _____ Occupation _____

Examiner _____

I. Health History

	No	Yes, explain
1. Any **difficulty seeing** or blurring?		
2. Any eye **pain**?		
3. Any history of **crossed eyes**?		
4. Any **redness** or **swelling** in eyes?		
5. Any **watering** or **tearing**?		
6. Any **injury** or **surgery** to eye?		
7. Ever tested for **glaucoma**?		
8. Wear **glasses** or **contact lenses**?		
9. Ever had vision tested?		
10. Taking any medications?		

II. Physical Examination

A. Test visual acuity
Snellen eye chart _____
Pocket vision screener for near vision _____

B. Test visual fields
Confrontation test _____

C. Inspect extraocular muscle function
Corneal light reflex _____
Cover test _____
Diagnostic positions test _____

D. Inspect external eye structures
General _____
Eyebrows _____
Eyelids and lashes _____
Eyeballs _____
Conjunctiva and sclera _____
Lacrimal gland, puncta _____

E. Inspect anterior eyeball structures
Cornea _____
Iris _____
Pupil size _____
Pupil direct and consensual light reflex _____
Accommodation _____

F. Inspect ocular fundus
Optic disc _____
Vessels _____
General background of fundus _____
Macula _____

REGIONAL WRITE-UP—EYES

Summarize your findings using the SOAP format.

Subjective (Reason for seeking care, health history)

Objective (Physical exam findings)

Record findings on diagram below

R   L

Assessment (Assessment of problem, diagnosis)

Plan (Diagnostic evaluation, follow-up care, teaching)

CHAPTER *15*

Ears

PURPOSE

This chapter helps you to learn the structure and function of the ears; to learn the methods of examination of hearing, external ear structures, and tympanic membrane using the otoscope; and to record the assessment accurately.

READING ASSIGNMENT

Jarvis, *Physical Examination and Health Assessment,* 4th ed., Chapter 15, pp. 341-370.

AUDIO-VISUAL ASSIGNMENT

Jarvis, *Saunders Video Assessment Series: Head, Eyes, and Ears*

GLOSSARY

Study the following terms after completing the reading assignment. You should be able to cover the definition on the right and define the term out loud.

Annulus .... outer fibrous rim encircling the eardrum

Atresia .... congenital absence or closure of ear canal

Cerumen .... yellow waxy material that lubricates and protects the ear canal

Cochlea .... inner ear structure containing the central hearing apparatus

Eustachian tube .... connects the middle ear with the nasopharynx and allows passage of air

Helix .... superior, posterior free rim of the pinna

Incus .... "anvil," middle of the 3 ossicles of the middle ear

Malleus .... "hammer," first of the 3 ossicles of the middle ear

Mastoid .... bony prominence of the skull located just behind the ear

Organ of Corti .... sensory organ of hearing

Otalgia .... pain in the ear

Otitis externa .... inflammation of the outer ear and ear canal

Otitis media .... inflammation of the middle ear and tympanic membrane

Otorrhea.................................... discharge from the ear

Pars flaccida .... small, slack, superior section of tympanic membrane

Pars tensa .... thick, taut, central/inferior section of tympanic membrane

Pinna .... auricle, or outer ear

Stapes... "stirrup," inner of the 3 ossicles of the middle ear

Tinnitus .... ringing in the ears

Tympanic membrane .... "eardrum," thin, translucent, oval membrane that stretches across the ear canal and separates the middle ear from the outer ear

Umbo .... knob of the malleus that shows through the tympanic membrane

Vertigo .... a spinning, twirling sensation

STUDY GUIDE

After completing the reading assignment and the audio-visual assignment, you should be able to answer the following questions in the spaces provided.

1. List the 3 functions of the middle ear.

2. Contrast 2 pathways of hearing.

3. Differentiate among the types of hearing loss, and give examples.

4. Relate the anatomic differences that place the infant at greater risk for middle ear infections.

5. Describe these tests of hearing acuity: voice test; Weber test; Rinne test.

6. Explain the positioning of normal ear alignment in the child.

7. Define *otosclerosis* and *presbycusis.*

8. Contrast the motions used to straighten the ear canal when using the otoscope with an infant versus an adult.

9. Describe the appearance of these nodules that could be present on the external ear: Darwin's tubercle; sebaceous cyst; tophi; chondrodermatitis; keloid; carcinoma.

10. Describe the appearance of these conditions that could appear in the ear canal: osteoma; exostosis; furuncle; polyp; foreign body.

11. List the indications of the following descriptions of the appearance of the eardrum: yellow-amber color _____; pearly gray color _____; air-fluid level _____; distorted light reflex _____; red color _____; dense white areas _____; oval dark areas _____; black or white dots on drum _____; blue drum _____.

12. List the findings that commonly appear during the Weber test and the Rinne test for:

    Conductive hearing loss _____

    _____

    Sensorineural loss _____

    _____

13. Fill in the labels indicated on the following illustrations.

REVIEW QUESTIONS

This test is for you and is intended to check your own mastery of the content. Answers are provided in Appendix A.

1. Using the otoscope, the tympanic membrane is visualized. The color of a normal membrane is:

   a) deep pink.
   b) creamy white.
   c) pearly gray.
   d) dependent upon the ethnicity of the individual.

2. Sensorineural hearing loss may be related to:

   a) a gradual nerve degeneration.
   b) foreign bodies.
   c) impacted cerumen.
   d) perforated tympanic membrane.

3. Prior to examining the ear with the otoscope, the _____ should be palpated for tenderness.

   a) helix, external auditory meatus, and lobule
   b) mastoid process, tympanic membrane, and malleus
   c) pinna, pars flaccida, and antitragus
   d) pinna, tragus, and mastoid process

4. During the otoscopic examination of a child less than 3 years of age, the examiner:

   a) pulls the pinna up and back.
   b) pulls the pinna down.
   c) holds the pinna gently but firmly in its normal position.
   d) tilts the head slightly toward the examiner.

5. While viewing with the otoscope, the examiner instructs the person to hold the nose and swallow. During this maneuver, the eardrum should:

   a) flutter.
   b) retract.
   c) bulge.
   d) remain immobile.

6. To differentiate between air conduction and bone conduction hearing loss, the examiner would perform:

   a) Weber's test.
   b) the Romberg test.
   c) the Rinne test.
   d) the whisper test.

7. In examining the ear of an adult, the canal is straightened by pulling the auricle:

   a) down and forward.
   b) down and back.
   c) up and back.
   d) up and forward.

8. Darwin's tubercle is:

   a) an overgrowth of scar tissue.
   b) a blocked sebaceous gland.
   c) a sign of gout called tophi.
   d) a congenital, painless nodule at the helix.

9. When the ear is being examined with the otoscope, the patient's head should be:

   a) tilted toward the examiner.
   b) titled away from the examiner.
   c) as vertical as possible.
   d) tilted down.

10. The hearing receptors are located in the:

   a) vestibule.
   b) semicircular canals.
   c) middle ear.
   d) cochlea.

11. The sensation of vertigo is the result of:

    a) otitis media.
    b) pathology in the semicircular canals.
    c) pathology in the cochlea.
    d) 4th cranial nerve damage.

12. A common cause of a conductive hearing loss is:

    a) impacted cerumen.
    b) acute rheumatic fever.
    c) a CVA.
    d) otitis externa.

13. In the Rinne test, the 2 to 1 ratio refers to:

    a) the loudness of the tone heard by the two ears.
    b) the lengths of time until the patient stops hearing the tone by air conduction and by bone conduction.
    c) the lengths of time until the patient no longer hears the tone and the examiner no longer hears the tone.
    d) the examiner hearing the tone twice as long as the patient hears it.

14. Upon examination of the tympanic membrane, visualization of which of the following findings indicates the infection of acute purulent otitis media?

    a) absent light reflex, bluish drum, oval dark areas
    b) absent light reflex, reddened drum, bulging drum
    c) oval dark areas on drum
    d) absent light reflex, air-fluid level or bubbles behind drum
    e) retracted drum, very prominent landmarks

15. In examining a young adult woman, you observe her tympanic membrane to be yellow in color. You suspect she has:

    a) serum in the middle ear.
    b) blood in the middle ear.
    c) infection of the drumhead.
    d) jaundice.

16. Risk reduction for acute otitis media includes:

    a) use of pacifiers.
    b) increasing group day care.
    c) avoiding breast-feeding.
    d) eliminating smoking in the house and car.

SKILLS LABORATORY/CLINICAL SETTING

You are now ready for the clinical component of the ear examination. The purpose of the clinical component is to practice the steps of the ear examination on a peer in the skills laboratory or on a patient in the clinical setting. The use of the otoscope is somewhat easier than the use of the ophthalmoscope; however, you still must be sure you are holding the instrument correctly. Holding the otoscope in an "upside down" position seems awkward at first, but it is important in order to make sure the otoscope tip does not cause pain to the delicate parts of the ear canal. Have someone correct your positioning before you insert the instrument.

CLINICAL OBJECTIVES

1. Collect a health history related to pertinent signs and symptoms of the ear system.

2. Describe the appearance of the normal outer ear and external ear canal.

3. Describe and demonstrate the correct technique of an otoscopic examination.

4. Describe and perform tests for hearing acuity.

5. Systematically describe the normal tympanic membrane including position, color, and landmarks.

6. Record the history and physical examination findings accurately, reach an assessment about the health state, and develop a plan of care.

INSTRUCTIONS

Prepare the examination setting and gather your equipment. Make certain the otoscope light is bright and batteries are freshly charged. Wash your hands. Practice the steps of the exam on a peer in the skills laboratory, giving appropriate instructions as you proceed. Record your findings using the regional write-up sheet that follows. The front of the page is intended as a worksheet; the back of the page is intended for your narrative summary recording using the SOAP format.

NOTES

REGIONAL WRITE-UP—EARS

Date _____

Patient _____ Age _____ Sex _____ Occupation _____

Examiner _____

I. Health History

	No	Yes, explain
1. Any **earache** or ear pain?	_____	_____
2. Any ear **infections**?	_____	_____
3. Any **discharge** from ears?	_____	_____
4. Any **hearing loss**?	_____	_____
5. Any **loud noises** at home or job?	_____	_____
6. Any **ringing** or buzzing in ears?	_____	_____
7. Ever felt **vertigo** (spinning)?	_____	_____
8. How do you clean your ears?	_____

II. Physical Examination

A. Inspect and palpate external ear

Size and shape _____

Skin condition _____

Tenderness _____

External auditory meatus _____

B. Inspect using the otoscope

External canal _____

Tympanic membrane _____

    Color and characteristics _____

    Position _____

    Integrity of membrane _____

C. Test hearing acuity

Voice test _____

Weber test _____

Rinne test _____

REGIONAL WRITE-UP—EARS

Summarize your findings using the SOAP format.

Subjective (Reason for seeking care, health history)

Objective (Physical exam findings)   Record findings on diagram below.

Assessment (Assessment of health state or problem, diagnosis)

Plan (Diagnostic evaluation, follow-up care, patient teaching)

CHAPTER 16

Nose, Mouth, and Throat

PURPOSE

This chapter helps you to learn the structure and function of the nose, mouth, and throat; to learn the methods of inspection and palpation of these structures; and to record the assessment accurately.

READING ASSIGNMENT

Jarvis, *Physical Examination and Health Assessment*, 4th ed., Chapter 16, pp. 371-406.

AUDIO-VISUAL ASSIGNMENT

Jarvis, *Saunders Video Assessment Series: Nose, Mouth, Throat, and Neck*

GLOSSARY

Study the following terms after completing the reading assignment. You should be able to cover the definition on the right and define the term out loud.

Aphthous ulcers .... "canker sores"—small, painful, round ulcers in the oral mucosa of unknown cause

Buccal .... pertaining to the cheek

Candidiasis .... (moniliasis) white, cheesy, curdlike patch on buccal mucosa due to superficial fungal infection

Caries .... decay in the teeth

Crypts .... indentations on surface of tonsils

Cheilitis .... red, scaling, shallow, painful fissures at corners of mouth

Choanal atresia .... closure of nasal cavity due to congenital septum between nasal cavity and pharynx

Epistaxis .... nosebleed, usually from anterior septum

Epulis .... nontender, fibrous nodule of the gum

Fordyce's granules .... small, isolated, white or yellow papules on oral mucosa

Gingivitis .... red swollen gum margins that bleed easily

Herpes simplex .... "cold sores"—clear vesicles with red base, which evolve into pustules, usually at lip-skin junction

Koplik's spots .... small, blue-white spots with red halo over oral mucosa; early sign of measles

Leukoplakia .... chalky white, thick raised patch on sides of tongue; precancerous

Malocclusion .... upper or lower dental arches out of alignment

Papillae .... rough bumpy elevation on dorsal surface of tongue

Parotid glands .... pair of salivary glands in the cheeks in front of the ears

Pharyngitis .... inflammation of the throat

Plaque .... soft whitish debris on teeth

Polyp .... smooth, pale gray nodules in the nasal cavity due to chronic allergic rhinitis

Rhinitis .... red swollen inflammation of nasal mucosa

Thrush .... oral candidiasis in the newborn

Turbinate .... one of 3 bony projections into nasal cavity

Uvula .... free projection hanging down from the middle of the soft palate

STUDY GUIDE

After completing the reading assignment and the audio-visual assignment, you should be able to answer the following questions in the spaces provided.

1. Name the functions of the nose.

2. Describe the size and components of the nasal cavity.

3. List the 4 sets of paranasal sinuses and describe their function.

4. List the 3 pairs of salivary glands, including their location and the locations of their duct openings.

5. Following tooth loss in the middle or older adult, describe the consequences of chewing with the remaining maloccluded teeth.

6. Describe the appearance of a deviated nasal septum and a perforated septum.

7. Describe the appearance of a torus palatinus and explain its significance.

8. Contrast the physical appearance and clinical significance of: leukoedema; candidiasis; leukoplakia; Fordyce's granules.

9. List the 4-point grading scale for the size of tonsils.

10. Describe the appearance and clinical significance of these findings in the infant: sucking tubercle; Epstein's pearls; Bednar's aphthae.

11. Contrast the appearance of nasal turbinates versus nasal polyps.

12. Describe the appearance and clinical significance of these findings on the tongue: ankyloglossia; fissured tongue; geographic tongue; black hairy tongue; macroglossia.

13. In the space below, sketch a cleft palate and a bifid uvula.

14. Describe the appearance of oral Kaposi's sarcoma.

ASSESSMENT VIDEO CRITICAL THINKING QUESTIONS

Discussion answers to these questions are in the Instructor's Manual for *Physical Examination and Health Assessment*, 4th ed.

1. How may oral self-care affect mouth examination findings?

2. Describe abnormal findings that may be found during inspection of the internal nose.

3. How do mouth examination findings vary among darkly pigmented people?

Fill in the labels indicated on the following illustrations.

LEFT LATERAL WALL-NASAL CAVITY

REVIEW QUESTIONS

This test is for you and is intended to check your own mastery of the content. Answers are provided in Appendix A.

1. The most common site of nosebleeds is:

   a) the turbinates.
   b) the columellae.
   c) Kiesselbach's plexus.
   d) the meatus.

2. The sinuses that are accessible to examination are the:

   a) ethmoid and sphenoid.
   b) frontal and ethmoid.
   c) maxillary and sphenoid.
   d) frontal and maxillary sinuses.

3. The frenulum is:

   a) the midline fold of tissue that connects the tongue to the floor of the mouth.
   b) the anterior border of the oral cavity.
   c) the arching roof of the mouth.
   d) the free projection hanging down from the middle of the soft palate.

4. The largest salivary gland is located:

   a) within the cheeks in front of the ear.
   b) beneath the mandible at the angle of the jaw.
   c) within the floor of the mouth under the tongue.
   d) at the base of the tongue.

5. A 70-year-old woman complains of dry mouth. The most frequent cause of this problem is:

   a) the aging process.
   b) related to medications she may be taking.
   c) the use of dentures.
   d) related to a diminished sense of smell.

6. Because of a history of headache, the examiner uses transillumination to assess for an inflamed sinus. The findings in a healthy individual would be:

   a) a diffuse red glow.
   b) no transillumination.
   c) findings vary with ethnicity of the person.
   d) light visible in the nares through a speculum.

7. During an inspection of the nares, a deviated septum is noted. The best action is to:

   a) request a consultation with an ear, nose, and throat specialist.
   b) document the deviation in the medical record in case the person needs to be suctioned.
   c) teach the person what to do if a nosebleed should occur.
   d) explore further because polyps frequently accompany a deviated septum.

8. Oral malignancies are most likely to develop:

   a) on the soft palate.
   b) on the tongue.
   c) in the buccal cavity.
   d) under the tongue.

9. In a medical record, the tonsils are graded as 3 +. The tonsils would be:

   a) visible.
   b) halfway between the tonsillar pillars and uvula.
   c) touching the uvula.
   d) touching each other.

10. The function of the nasal turbinates is to:

   a) warm the inhaled air.
   b) detect odors.
   c) stimulate tear formation.
   d) lighten the weight of the skull bones.

11. The opening of an adult's parotid gland (Stensen's duct) is opposite the:

   a) lower 2nd molar.
   b) lower incisors.
   c) upper incisors.
   d) upper 2nd molar.

12. A nasal polyp may be distinguished from the nasal turbinates for 3 of the following reasons. Which reason is *false*?

   a) The polyp is highly vascular.
   b) The polyp is movable.
   c) The polyp is pale gray in color.
   d) The polyp is nontender.

SKILLS LABORATORY/CLINICAL SETTING

You are now ready for the clinical component of the nose, mouth, and throat examination. The purpose of the clinical component is to practice the steps of the examination on a peer in the skills laboratory or on a patient in the clinical setting and to achieve the following.

CLINICAL OBJECTIVES

1. Inspect the external nose.

2. Demonstrate use of the otoscope and nasal attachment to inspect the structures of the nasal cavity.

3. Demonstrate knowledge of infection control practices during inspection and palpation of structures of the mouth and pharynx.

4. Record the history and physical examination findings accurately, reach an assessment of the health state, and develop a plan of care.

INSTRUCTIONS

Prepare the examination setting and gather your equipment. Wash your hands. Practice the steps of the exam on a peer in the skills laboratory, giving appropriate instructions as you proceed. Record your findings using the regional write-up sheet that follows. The front of the page is intended as a worksheet; the back of the page is intended for your narrative summary recording using the SOAP format.

REGIONAL WRITE-UP—NOSE, MOUTH, AND THROAT

Date _____

Patient _____ Age _____ Sex _____ Occupation _____

Examiner _____

I. Health History

A. Nose   No | Yes, explain

    1. Any nasal **discharge**?

    2. Unusually frequent or severe colds?

    3. Any **sinus pain** or sinusitis?

    4. Any **trauma** or injury to nose?

    5. Any **nosebleeds**? How often?

    6. Any **allergies** or hay fever?

    7. Any change in sense of smell?

B. Mouth and throat

    1. Any **sores** in mouth, tongue?

    2. Any **sore throat**? How often?

    3. Any **bleeding gums**?

    4. Any **toothache**?

    5. Any **hoarseness,** voice change?

    6. Any difficulty **swallowing**?

    7. Any change in sense of taste?

    8. Do you smoke? How much/day?

    9. Tell me about usual dental care.

II. Physical Examination

A. Inspect and palpate the nose

    Symmetry _____

    Deformity, asymmetry, inflammation _____

    Test patency of each nostril _____

    Using a nasal speculum, note:

       Color of nasal mucosa _____

       Discharge, foreign body _____

       Septum: deviation, perforation, bleeding _____

       Turbinates: color, swelling, exudate, polyps _____

B. Palpate the sinus area

    Frontal _____

    Maxillary _____

    Transillumination (if indicated) _____

C. Inspect the mouth

    Lips _____

    Teeth and gums _____

    Buccal mucosa _____

    Palate and uvula _____

D. Inspect the throat
  Tonsils: condition and grade _____
  Pharyngeal wall _____
  Any breath odor _____

REGIONAL WRITE-UP—NOSE, MOUTH, AND THORAT

Summarize your findings using the SOAP format.

Subjective (Reason for seeking care, health history)

Objective (Physical exam findings)

Record findings on diagram below.

Assessment (Assessment of health state or problem, diagnosis)

Plan (Diagnostic evaluation, follow-up care, patient teaching)

CHAPTER 17

Breasts and Regional Lymphatics

PURPOSE

This chapter helps you to learn the structure and function of the breast, to understand the rationale and methods of examination of the breast, to accurately record the assessment, and to teach breast self-examination.

READING ASSIGNMENT

Jarvis, *Physical Examination and Health Assessment*, 4th ed., Chapter 17, pp. 407-436.

AUDIO-VISUAL ASSIGNMENT

Jarvis, *Saunders Video Series, Physical Examination and Health Assessment: Breasts and Regional Lymphatics*

GLOSSARY

Study the following terms after completing the reading assignment. You should be able to cover the definition on the right and define the term out loud.

Alveoli .... smallest structure of mammary gland

Areola .... darkened area surrounding nipple

Colostrum .... thin, yellow fluid, precursor of milk, secreted for a few days after birth

Cooper's ligaments .... suspensory ligament, fibrous bands extending from the inner breast surface to the chest wall muscles

Fibroadenoma .... benign breast mass

Gynecomastia .... excessive breast development in the male

Intraductal papilloma .... serosanguinous nipple discharge

Inverted .... nipples that are depressed or invaginated

Lactiferous .... conveying milk

Mastitis .... inflammation of the breast

Montgomery's glands .... sebaceous glands in the areola, secrete protective lipid during lactation; also called tubercles of Montgomery

Paget's disease .... intraductal carcinoma in the breast

Peau d'orange .... orange-peel appearance of breast due to edema

Retraction .... dimple or pucker on the skin

Striae .... atrophic pink, purple, or white linear streaks on the breasts, associated with pregnancy, excessive weight gain, or rapid growth during adolescence

Supernumerary nipple .... minute extra nipple along the embryonic milk line

Tail of Spence .... extension of breast tissue into the axilla

STUDY GUIDE

After completing the reading assignment and the audio-visual assignment, you should be able to answer the following questions in the spaces provided.

1. Identify appropriate history questions to ask regarding the breast exam.

2. Describe the anatomy of the breast.

3. Correlate changes in the female breast with normal developmental stages.

4. Describe the components of the breast exam.

5. List points to include in teaching the breast self-exam.

6. Explain the significance of a supernumerary nipple/breast.

7. Differentiate between the female and male examination procedure and findings.

8. Discuss pathologic changes that may occur in the breast:

    Benign breast disease

    Abscess

    Acute mastitis

    Fibroadenoma

    Cancer

    Paget's disease

9. List and describe the characteristics to consider when a mass is noted in the breast.

10. Define gynecomastia.

11. Recall additional diagnostic techniques used for diagnosis of breast lesions.

12. List the high-risk and moderate-risk factors that increase the usual risk of breast cancer.

ASSESSMENT VIDEO CRITICAL THINKING QUESTIONS

Discussion answers to these questions are in the Instructor's Manual for *Physical Examination and Health Assessment*, 4th ed.

1. How do breast assessment findings differ between older women and younger adult women?

2. How should you modify breast palpation in a woman with large, pendulous breasts?

3. Which conditions may be associated with a breast lump? Nipple rash? Enlarged axillary lymph nodes?

Fill in the labels on the following diagrams.

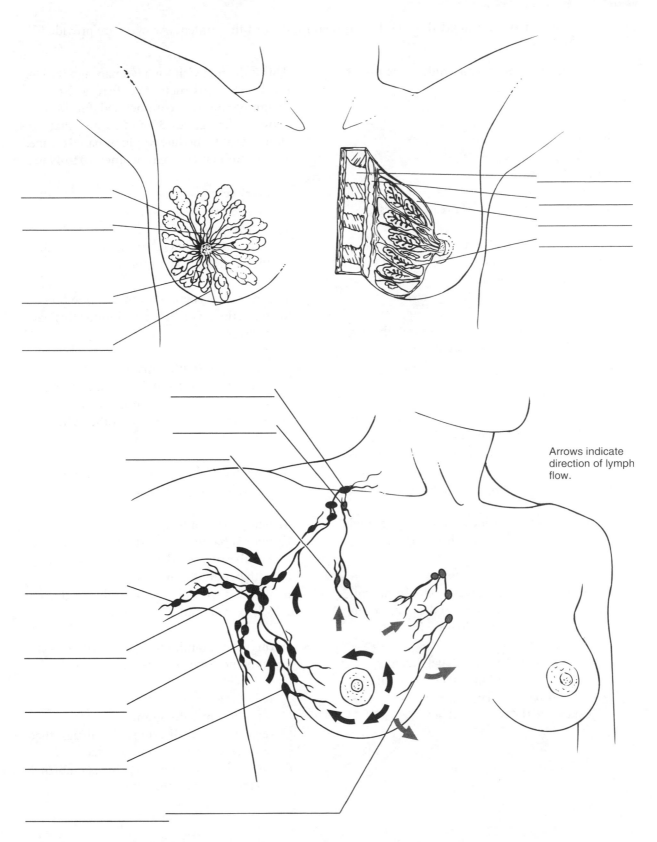

Arrows indicate direction of lymph flow.

REVIEW QUESTIONS

This test is for you and is intended to check your own mastery of the content. Answers are provided in Appendix A.

1. The reservoirs for storing milk in the breast are:

   a) lobules.
   b) alveoli.
   c) Montgomery's glands.
   d) lactiferous sinuses.

2. The most common site of breast tumors is:

   a) upper inner quadrant.
   b) upper outer quadrant.
   c) lower inner quadrant.
   d) lower outer quadrant.

3. During a visit for a school physical, the 13-year-old girl being examined questions the asymmetry of her breasts. The best response is:

   a) "One breast may grow faster than the other during development."
   b) "I will give you a referral for a mammogram."
   c) "You will probably have fibrocystic disease when you are older."
   d) "This may be an indication of hormonal imbalance. We will check again in 6 months."

4. When teaching the breast self-exam, you would inform the woman that the best time to conduct breast self-examination is:

   a) at the onset of the menstrual period.
   b) on the 14th day of the menstrual cycle.
   c) on the 4th to 7th day of the cycle.
   d) just before the menstrual period.

5. This is the first visit for a woman, age 38. The practitioner instructs her that a baseline mammogram is recommended for women between the ages of 35 and 39 and that the clinical exam schedule would be based on age. The recommendation for women 40 to 49 is:

   a) every year.
   b) every 2 years.
   c) twice a year.
   d) only the baseline exam is needed unless the woman has symptoms.

6. The examiner is going to inspect the breasts for retraction. The best position for this part of the exam is:

   a) lying supine with arms at the sides.
   b) leaning forward with hands outstretched.
   c) sitting with hand pushing onto hips.
   d) one arm at the side, the other arm elevated.

7. A bimanual technique may be the preferred approach for a woman:

   a) who is pregnant.
   b) who is having the first breast exam by a health care provider.
   c) with pendulous breasts.
   d) who has felt a change in the breast during self examination.

8. During the examination of a 70-year-old man, you note gynecomastia. You would:

   a) refer for a biopsy.
   b) refer for a mammogram.
   c) review the medications for drugs that have gynecomastia as a side effect.
   d) proceed with the exam. This is a normal part of the aging process.

9. During a breast examination, you detect a mass. Identify the description that is most consistent with cancer rather than benign breast disease.

   a) round, firm, well demarcated
   b) irregular, poorly defined, fixed
   c) rubbery, mobile, tender
   d) lobular, clear margins, negative skin retraction

10. During the examination of the breasts of a pregnant woman, you would expect to find:

    a) peau d'orange.
    b) nipple retraction.
    c) a unilateral, obvious venous pattern.
    d) a blue vascular pattern over both breasts.

11. Which of the following women should *not* be referred to a physician for further evaluation?

    a) a 26-year-old with multiple nodules palpated in each breast
    b) a 48-year-old who has a 6-month history of reddened and sore left nipple and areolar area
    c) a 25-year-old with asymmetrical breasts and inversion of nipples since adolescence
    d) a 64-year-old with ulcerated area at tip of right nipple, no masses, tenderness, or lymph nodes palpated

12. Breast asymmetry:

    a) increases with age and parity.
    b) may be normal.
    c) indicates a neoplasm.
    d) is accompanied by enlarged axillary lymph nodes.

13. Any lump found in the breast should be referred for further evaluation. A benign lesion will usually have 3 of the following characteristics. Which one is characteristic of a *malignant* lesion?

    a) soft
    b) well-defined margins
    c) freely movable
    d) irregular shape

14. Gynecomastia is:

    a) enlargement of the male breast.
    b) presence of "mast" cells in the male breast.
    c) cancer of the male breast.
    d) presence of supernumerary breast on the male chest.

15. Which is the first physical change associated with puberty in girls?

    a) areolar elevation
    b) breast bud development
    c) height spurt
    d) pubic hair development
    e) menarche

SKILLS LABORATORY/CLINICAL SETTING

You are now ready for the clinical component of the breast assessment. The purpose of the clinical component is to practice the steps of the assessment on a peer in the skills laboratory and to achieve the following.

CLINICAL OBJECTIVES

1. Demonstrate knowledge of the symptoms related to the breasts and axillae by obtaining a health history.

2. Perform inspection and palpation of the breasts, with the woman in sitting and supine positions, using proper technique and providing appropriate draping.

3. Teach the breast self-exam to a woman or list the points to include in teaching the breast self-exam.

4. Record the history and physical exam findings accurately, reach an assessment of the health state, and develop a plan of care.

INSTRUCTIONS

Practice the steps of the breast exam on a peer or on a woman in the clinical area. Record your findings on the regional write-up sheet that follows. The front of the page is intended as a worksheet; the back of the page is intended for your narrative summary recording using the SOAP format.

Note the student performance checklist that follows the regional write-up sheet. It lists the essential behaviors you should display as an examiner, and it may be used by your clinical instructor to evaluate your clinical teaching of breast self-examination.

NOTES

REGIONAL WRITE-UP—BREASTS AND AXILLAE

Date _____

Patient _____ Age _____ Sex _____ Occupation _____
Examiner _____

I. Health History

	No	Yes, explain
1. Any **pain** or tenderness in breasts?	_____	_____
2. Any **lump** or thickening in breasts?	_____	_____
3. Any **discharge** from nipples?	_____	_____
4. Any **rash** on breasts?	_____	_____
5. Any **swelling** in the breasts?	_____	_____
6. Any **trauma** or injury to breasts?	_____	_____
7. Any **history** of breast disease?	_____	_____
8. Ever had **surgery** on breasts?	_____	_____
9. Ever been taught breast self-exam?	_____	_____
10. Ever had mammography?	_____	_____

II. Physical Examination

A. Inspection

1. Breasts

   Symmetry _____

   Skin color and condition _____

   Texture _____

   Lesions _____

2. Areolae and nipples

   Shape _____

   Direction _____

   Surface characteristics _____

   Discharge _____

3. Response to arm movement _____

4. Axillae _____

B. Palpation

1. Breasts

   Texture _____

   Masses _____

   Tenderness _____

2. Areolae and nipples

   Masses _____

   Discharge _____

3. Axillae and lymph nodes

   Size _____

   Shape _____

   Consistency _____

   Mobility _____

   Discrete or matted _____

   Tenderness _____

C. Teach breast self-exam

REGIONAL WRITE-UP—BREASTS AND AXILLAE

Summarize your findings using the SOAP format.
Subjective (Reason for seeking care, health history)

Objective (Physical exam findings)

Record findings on diagram below.

Assessment (Assessment of health state or problem, diagnosis)

Plan (Diagnostic evaluation, follow-up care, teaching)

PERFORMANCE CHECKLIST

TEACHING BREAST SELF-EXAMINATION (BSE)

	S	U	Comments
I. Cognitive 1. Explain: a. Why breasts are examined			
(1) in the shower			
(2) before a mirror			
(3) supine with pillow under side of breast being examined			
b. who should do breast exam			
c. frequency of breast exam			
d. best time of the month to do breast exam and rationale			
2. State the area of breast where most lumps are found			
3. Give two reasons a person may not report significant findings to the health care provider			
II. Performance			
1. Explains to woman need for BSE			
2. Instructs woman on technique of BSE by: a. inspecting and bilaterally comparing breasts in front of mirror			
b. palpating breast in a systemic manner, using pads of three fingers and with woman's arm raised overhead			
c. palpating tail of Spence and axilla			
d. gently compressing nipples			
3. Instructs woman to report unusual findings to the physician at once			

CHAPTER 18

Thorax and Lungs

PURPOSE

This chapter helps you to learn the structure and function of the thorax and lungs, to understand the methods of examination of the respiratory system, to identify lung sounds that are normal, to describe the characteristics of adventitious lung sounds, and to accurately record the assessment. At the end of this unit you will be able to perform a complete physical examination of the respiratory system.

READING ASSIGNMENT

Jarvis, *Physical Examination and Health Assessment*, 4th ed., Chapter 18, pp. 437-482.

AUDIO-VISUAL ASSIGNMENT

Jarvis, *Saunders Video Series, Physical Examination and Health Assessment: Thorax and Lungs.*

GLOSSARY

Study the following terms after completing the reading assignment. You should be able to cover the definition on the right and define the term out loud.

Alveoli.. functional units of the lung; the thin-walled chambers surrounded by networks of capillaries that are the site of respiratory exchange of carbon dioxide and oxygen

Angle of Louis............................ manubriosternal angle, the articulation of the manubrium and body of the sternum, continuous with the second rib

Apnea.. cessation of breathing

Asthma .... an abnormal respiratory condition associated with allergic hypersensitivity to certain inhaled allergens, characterized by bronchospasm, wheezing, and dyspnea

Atelectasis .... an abnormal respiratory condition characterized by collapsed, shrunken, deflated section of alveoli

Bradypnea .... slow breathing, < 10 breaths per minute, regular rate

Bronchiole .... one of the smaller respiratory passageways into which the segmental bronchi divide

Bronchitis .... inflammation of the bronchi with partial obstruction of bronchi due to excessive mucus secretion

Bronchophony .... the spoken voice sound heard through the stethoscope, which sounds soft, muffled, and indistinct over normal lung tissue

Bronchovesicular .... the normal breath sound heard over major bronchi, characterized by moderate pitch and an equal duration of inspiration and expiration

Chronic obstructive pulmonary disease (COPD) ..... a functional category of abnormal respiratory conditions characterized by airflow obstruction, e.g., emphysema, chronic bronchitis

Cilia .... millions of hairlike cells lining the tracheobronchial tree

Consolidation .... the solidification of portions of lung tissue as it fills up with infectious exudate, as in pneumonia

Crackles .... (rales) abnormal, discontinuous, adventitious lung sounds heard on inspiration

Crepitus .... coarse crackling sensation palpable over the skin when air abnormally escapes from the lung and enters the subcutaneous tissue

Dead space .... passageways that transport air but are not available for gaseous exchange, e.g., trachea and bronchi

Dyspnea .... difficult, labored breathing

Egophony .... the voice sound of "eeeeee" heard through the stethoscope

Emphysema .... the chronic obstructive pulmonary disease characterized by enlargement of alveoli distal to terminal bronchioles

Fissure .... the narrow crack dividing the lobes of the lungs

Fremitus .... a palpable vibration from the spoken voice felt over the chest wall

Friction rub .... a coarse, grating, adventitious lung sound heard when the pleurae are inflamed

Hypercapnia .... (hypercarbia) increased levels of carbon dioxide in the blood

Hyperventilation .... increased rate and depth of breathing

Hypoxemia .... decreased level of oxygen in the blood

Intercostal space .... space between the ribs

Kussmaul's respiration .... a type of hyperventilation that occurs with diabetic ketoacidosis

Orthopnea .... ability to breathe easily only in an upright position

Paroxysmal nocturnal dyspnea .... sudden awakening from sleeping with shortness of breath

Percussion .... striking over the chest wall with short sharp blows of the fingers in order to determine the size and density of the underlying organ

Pleural effusion .... abnormal fluid between the layers of the pleura

Rhonchi .... low-pitched, musical, snoring, adventitious lung sound caused by air-flow obstruction from secretions

Tachypnea .... rapid shallow breathing, > 24 breaths per minute

Vesicular .... the soft, low-pitched, normal breath sounds heard over peripheral lung fields

Vital capacity .... the amount of air, following maximal inspiration, that can be exhaled

Wheeze .... high-pitched, musical, squeaking adventitious lung sound

Whispered pectoriloquy .... a whispered phrase heard through the stethoscope that sounds faint and inaudible over normal lung tissue

Xiphoid process .... sword-shaped lower tip of the sternum

STUDY GUIDE

After completing the reading assignment and the audio-visual assignment, you should be able to answer the following questions in the spaces provided.

1. List the questions to obtain a health history for the respiratory system.

2. Describe the pleura and its function.

3. List the structures that compose the respiratory dead space.

4. Summarize the mechanics of respiration.

5. List the elements included in the inspection of the respiratory system.

6. Discuss the significance of a "barrel chest."

7. List and describe common thoracic deformities.

8. List and describe 3 types of normal breath sounds.

9. Define 2 types of adventitious breath sounds.

10. The manubriosternal angle is also called _____.

    Why is it a useful landmark?

11. How many degrees in the normal costal angle? _____.

12. When comparing the anterior-posterior diameter of the chest to the transverse diameter, what is the expected ratio?

What is the significance of this?

13. What is tripod position?

14. List 3 factors that affect normal intensity of tactile fremitus.

1.

2.

3.

15. During percussion, which sound would you expect to predominate over normal lung tissue?

16. Normal findings for diaphragmatic excursion are:

17. List 5 factors that can cause extraneous noise during auscultation.

1.

2.

3.

4.

5.

18. Describe the 3 types of normal breath sounds:

Name	Location	Description

ASSESSMENT VIDEO CRITICAL THINKING QUESTIONS

Discussion answers to these questions are in the Instructor's Manual for *Physical Examination and Health Assessment*, 4th ed.

1. Which conditions are associated with a productive cough?

2. Describe the characteristics of the following adventitious sounds: fine crackles, coarse crackles, wheezes, and rhonchi.

3. What assessment findings are normal variations in a pregnant woman?

4. Which nursing diagnoses are most appropriate for a person with wheezes, dyspnea, and tachypnea?

Fill in the labels indicated on the following illustrations.

Draw in the lobes of the lungs and label their landmarks on the following two illustrations.

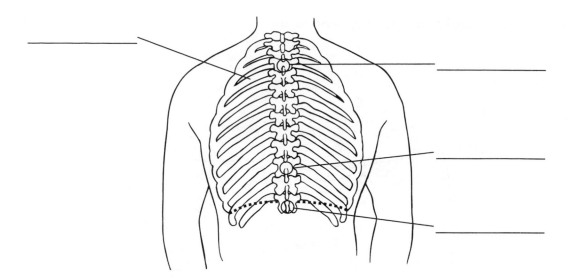

REVIEW QUESTIONS

This test is for you and is intended to check your own mastery of the content. Answers are provided in Appendix A.

1. The manubriosternal angle is:

   a) the articulation of the manubrium and the body of the sternum.
   b) a hollow, U-shaped depression just above the sternum.
   c) also known as the breastbone.
   d) a term synonymous with costochondral junction.

2. Select the correct description of the left lung.

   a) narrower than the right lung with three lobes
   b) narrower than the right with two lobes
   c) wider than the right lung with two lobes
   d) shorter than the right with three lobes

3. Some conditions have a cough with characteristic timing. The cough associated with chronic bronchitis is best described as:

   a) continuous throughout the day.
   b) productive cough for at least 3 months of the year for 2 years in a row.
   c) occurring in the afternoon/evening because of exposure to irritants at work.
   d) occurring in the early morning.

4. Symmetric chest expansion is best confirmed by:

   a) placing hands on the posterolateral chest wall with thumbs at the level of T9 or T10, then sliding the hands up to pinch up a small fold of skin between the thumbs.
   b) inspection of the shape and configuration of the chest wall.
   c) placing the palmar surface of the fingers of one hand against the chest and having the person repeat the words "ninety-nine."
   d) percussion of the posterior chest.

5. Absence of diaphragmatic excursion occurs with:

   a) asthma.
   b) an unusually thick chest wall.
   c) pleural effusion or atelectasis of the lower lobes.
   d) age-related changes in the chest wall.

6. Auscultation of breath sounds is an important component of respiratory assessment. Select the most accurate description of this part of the examination.

   a) Hold the bell of the stethoscope against the chest wall, listen to the entire right field, then the entire left field.
   b) Hold the diaphragm of the stethoscope against the chest wall; listen to one full respiration in each location, being sure to do side-to-side comparisons.
   c) Listen from the apices to the bases of each lung field using the bell of the stethoscope.
   d) Select the bell or diaphragm depending upon the quality of sounds heard; listen for one respiration in each location, moving from side to side.

7. Select the best description of bronchovesicular breath sounds:

   a) high pitched, of longer duration on inspiration than expiration.
   b) moderate pitch, inspiration equal to expiration.
   c) low pitched, inspiration greater than expiration.
   d) rustling sound, like the wind in the trees.

8. After examining a patient, you make the following notation: Increased respiratory rate, chest expansion decreased on left side, dull to percussion over left lower lobe, breath sounds louder with fine crackles over left lower lobe. These findings are consistent with a diagnosis of:

   a) bronchitis.
   b) asthma.
   c) pleural effusion.
   d) lobar pneumonia.

9. Upon examining a patient's nails, you note that the angle of the nail base is > 160 degrees and that the nail base feels spongy to palpation. These findings are consistent with:

   a) adult respiratory distress syndrome.
   b) normal findings for the nails.
   c) chronic, congenital heart disease and COPD.
   d) atelectasis.

10. Upon examination of a patient, you note a coarse, low-pitched sound during both inspiration and expiration. This patient complains of pain with breathing. These findings are consistent with:

   a) fine crackles.
   b) wheezes.
   c) atelectatic crackles.
   d) pleural friction rub.

11. In order to use the technique of egophony, ask the patient to:

   a) take several deep breaths, then hold for 5 seconds.
   b) say "ee" each time the stethoscope is moved.
   c) repeat the phrase "ninety-nine" each time the stethoscope is moved.
   d) whisper a phrase as auscultation is performed.

12. When examining for tactile fremitus, it is important to:

   a) have the patient breathe quickly.
   b) ask the patient to cough.
   c) palpate the chest symmetrically.
   d) use the bell of the stethoscope.

13. The pulse oximeter measures:

   a) arterial oxygen saturation.
   b) venous oxygen saturation.
   c) combined saturation of arterial and venous blood.
   d) carboxyhemoglobin levels.

Match column A to column B.

Column A—lung borders

14. _____ apex

15. _____ base

16. _____ lateral left

17. _____ lateral right

18. _____ posterior apex

Column B—location

a. rests on the diaphragm

b. C7

c. sixth rib, midclavicular line

d. fifth intercostal

e. 3 to 4 cm above the inner third of the clavicles

Match column A to column B

Column A—configurations of the thorax

19. _____ normal chest

20. _____ barrel chest

21. _____ pectus excavatum

22. _____ pectus carinatum

23. _____ scoliosis

24. _____ kyphosis

Column B—description

a. anteroposterior = transverse diameter

b. exaggerated posterior curvature of thoracic spine

c. lateral, S–shaped curvature of the thoracic and lumbar spine

d. sunken sternum and adjacent cartilages

e. elliptical shape with an anteroposterior: transverse diameter in the ratio of 1 : 2

f. forward protrusion of the sternum with ribs sloping back at either side

SKILLS LABORATORY/CLINICAL SETTING

You are now ready for the clinical component of the respiratory system. The purpose of the clinical component is to practice the regional examination on a peer in the skills laboratory or on a patient in the clinical setting and to achieve the following.

CLINICAL OBJECTIVES

1. Demonstrate knowledge of the symptoms related to the respiratory system by obtaining a regional health history from a peer/patient.

2. Correctly locate anatomic landmarks on the thorax of a peer.

3. Using a grease pencil, and with peer's permission, draw lobes of the lungs on a peer's thorax.

4. Demonstrate correct techniques for inspection, palpation, percussion, and auscultation of the respiratory system.

5. Demonstrate the technique for estimation of diaphragmatic excursion.

6. Record the history and physical exam findings accurately, reach an assessment of the health state, and develop a plan of care.

INSTRUCTIONS

Gather your equipment. Wash your hands. Clean the stethoscope endpiece with an alcohol wipe. Practice the steps of the exam of the thorax and lungs on a peer or on a patient in the clinical area. Record your findings using the regional write-up sheet. The front of the sheet is intended as a worksheet; the back of the sheet is intended for a narrative summary using the SOAP format.

NOTES

REGIONAL WRITE-UP—THORAX AND LUNGS

Date _____

Patient _____ Age _____ Sex _____ Occupation _____

Examiner _____

I. Health History

	No	Yes, explain
1. Do you have a **cough**?		
2. Any shortness of **breath**?		
3. Any **chest pain** with breathing?		
4. Any **past history** of lung diseases?		
5. **Smoke** cigarettes? How many/day?		
6. Any living or work conditions that affect your breathing?		
7. Last Tb skin test, chest x-ray, flu vaccine?		

II. Physical Examination

A. Inspection
1. Thoracic cage _____
2. Respiratory rate and pattern _____
3. Skin _____
4. Person's position _____
5. Person's facial expression _____
6. Level of consciousness _____

B. Palpation
1. Confirm symmetrical chest expansion _____
2. Tactile fremitus _____
3. Detect any lumps, masses, tenderness _____
4. Trachea _____

C. Percussion
1. Determine percussion note that predominates over lung fields _____
2. Diaphragmatic excursion _____

D. Auscultation
1. Listen: posterior, lateral, anterior _____
2. Any abnormal breath sounds? _____
   If so, perform bronchophony, _____
   whispered pectoriloquy, _____
   egophony _____
3. Any adventitious sounds? _____

REGIONAL WRITE-UP—THORAX AND LUNGS

Summarize your findings using the SOAP format.

Subjective (Reason for seeking care, health history)

Objective (Physical exam findings)

Use the drawing to diagram your findings.

Assessment (Assessment of health state or problem, diagnosis)

Plan (Diagnostic evaluation, follow-up care, teaching)

CHAPTER *19*

Heart and Neck Vessels

PURPOSE

This chapter helps you to learn the structure and function of the heart, valves, and great vessels; to understand the cardiac cycle; to describe the heart sounds; to understand the rationale and methods of examination of the heart; and to accurately record the assessment. At the end of this unit you should be able to perform a complete assessment of the heart and neck vessels.

READING ASSIGNMENT

Jarvis, *Physical Examination and Health Assessment*, 4th ed., Chapter 19, pp. 483-532.

AUDIO-VISUAL ASSIGNMENT

Jarvis, *Saunders Video Series, Physical Examination and Health Assessment: Cardiovascular System: Heart and Neck Vessels*

GLOSSARY

Study the following terms after completing the reading assignment. You should be able to cover the definition on the right and define the term out loud.

Angina pectoris .... acute chest pain that occurs when myocardial demand exceeds its oxygen supply

Aortic regurgitation.................. (aortic insufficiency) incompetent aortic valve that allows backward flow of blood into left ventricle during diastole

Aortic stenosis .... calcification of aortic valve cusps that restricts forward flow of blood during systole

Aortic valve .... the left semilunar valve separating the left ventricle and the aorta

Apex of the heart .... tip of the heart pointing down toward the 5th left intercostal space

Apical impulse .... (point of maximal impulse, PMI) pulsation created as the left ventricle rotates against the chest wall during systole, normally at the 5th left intercostal space in the midclavicular line

Base of the heart .... broader area of heart's outline located at the 3rd right and left intercostal space

Bell (of the stethoscope) .... cup-shaped endpiece used for soft, low-pitched heart sounds

Bradycardia .... slow heart rate, < 50 beats per minute in the adult

Clubbing .... bulbous enlargement of distal phalanges of fingers and toes that occurs with chronic cyanotic heart and lung conditions

Coarctation of aorta .... severe narrowing of the descending aorta, a congenital heart defect

Cor pulmonale .... right ventricular hypertrophy and heart failure due to pulmonary hypertension

Cyanosis .... dusky blue mottling of the skin and mucous membranes due to excessive amount of reduced hemoglobin in the blood

Diaphragm (of the stethoscope) .... flat endpiece of the stethoscope used for hearing relatively high-pitched heart sounds

Diastole .... the heart's filling phase

Dyspnea .... difficult, labored breathing

Edema .... swelling of legs or dependent body part due to increased interstitial fluid

Erb's point .... traditional auscultatory area in the 3rd left intercostal space

First heart sound (S_1) .... occurs with closure of the atrioventricular (AV) valves signaling the beginning of systole

Fourth heart sound (S_4) .... (S_4 gallop; atrial gallop) very soft, low-pitched, ventricular filling sound that occurs in late diastole

Gallop rhythm .... the addition of a 3rd or a 4th heart sound makes the rhythm sound like the cadence of a galloping horse

Inching .... technique of moving the stethoscope incrementally across the precordium through the auscultatory areas while listening to the heart sounds

LVH (left ventricular hypertrophy) .... increase in thickness of myocardial wall that occurs when the heart pumps against chronic outflow obstruction, e.g., aortic stenosis

MCL (midclavicular line) .... imaginary vertical line bisecting the middle of the clavicle in each hemithorax

Mitral regurgitation .... (mitral insufficiency) incompetent mitral valve allows regurgitation of blood back into left atrium during systole

Mitral stenosis .... calcified mitral valve impedes forward flow of blood into left ventricle during diastole

Mitral valve .... left AV valve separating the left atria and ventricle

Palpitation .... uncomfortable awareness of rapid or irregular heart rate

Paradoxical splitting .... opposite of a normal split S_2 so that the split is heard in expiration, and in inspiration the sounds fuse to one sound

Pericardial friction rub .... high-pitched scratchy extracardiac sound heard when the precordium is inflamed

Physiologic splitting .... normal variation in S_2 heard as two separate components during inspiration

Precordium .... area of the chest wall overlying the heart and great vessels

Pulmonic regurgitation .... (pulmonic insufficiency) backflow of blood through incompetent pulmonic valve into the right ventricle

Pulmonic stenosis .... calcification of pulmonic valve that restricts forward flow of blood during systole

Pulmonic valve .... right semilunar valve separating the right ventricle and pulmonary artery

Second heart sound (S_2) .... occurs with closure of the semilunar valves, aortic and pulmonic, and signals the end of systole

Summation gallop .... abnormal mid-diastolic heart sound heard when both the pathologic S_3 and S_4 are present

Syncope .... temporary loss of consciousness due to decreased cerebral blood flow (fainting), caused by ventricular asystole, pronounced bradycardia, or ventricular fibrillation

Systole .... the heart's pumping phase

Tachycardia .... rapid heart rate, > 100 beats per minute in the adult

Third heart sound (S_3) .... soft, low-pitched, ventricular filling sound that occurs in early diastole (S_3 gallop) and may be an early sign of heart failure

Thrill .... palpable vibration on the chest wall accompanying severe heart murmur

Tricuspid valve .... right AV valve separating the right atria and ventricle

STUDY GUIDE

After completing the reading assignment and the audio-visual assignment, you should be able to answer the following questions in the spaces provided.

1. Define the apical impulse and describe its normal location, size, and duration.

Which *normal* variations may affect the location of the apical impulse?

Which *abnormal* conditions may affect the location of the apical impulse?

2. Explain the mechanism producing normal first and second heart sounds.

3. Describe the effect of respiration on the heart sounds.

4. Describe the characteristics of the first heart sound and its intensity at the apex of the heart and at the base.

Which conditions *increase* the intensity of S_1?

Which conditions *decrease* the intensity of S_1?

5. Describe the characteristics of the second heart sound and its intensity at the apex of the heart and at the base.

Which conditions *increase* the intensity of S_2?

Which conditions *decrease* the intensity of S_2?

6. Explain the physiologic mechanism for normal splitting of S_2 in the pulmonic valve area.

7. Define the third heart sound. When in the cardiac cycle does it occur? Describe its intensity, quality, location in which it is heard, and method of auscultation.

8. Differentiate a physiologic S_3 from a pathologic S_3.

9. Define the fourth heart sound. When in the cardiac cycle does it occur? Describe its intensity, quality, location in which it is heard, and method of auscultation.

10. Explain the position of the valves during each phase of the cardiac cycle.

11. Define venous pressure and jugular venous pulse.

12. Differentiate between the carotid artery pulsation and the jugular vein pulsation.

13. List the areas of questioning to address during the health history of the cardiovascular system.

14. Define bruit, and discuss what it indicates.

15. Define heave or lift, and discuss what it indicates.

16. State 4 guidelines to distinguish S_1 from S_2.

   1. _____

   2. _____

   3. _____

   4. _____

17. Define pulse deficit, and discuss what it indicates.

18. Define preload and afterload.

19. List the characteristics to explore when you hear a murmur, including the grading scale of murmurs.

20. Discuss the characteristics of an innocent or functional murmur.

ASSESSMENT VIDEO CRITICAL THINKING QUESTIONS

Discussion answers to these questions are in the Instructor's Manual for *Physical Examination and Health Assessment*, 4th ed.

1. What cardiac risk factors are important to explore during the health history? How do they affect cardiovascular function?

2. How would you modify your technique when assessing an older adult's neck vessels?

3. How do you describe sinus arrhythmia, and what does it signify?

4. What heart sounds should you expect to hear in a person with aortic stenosis?

Fill in the labels indicated on the following illustrations.

REVIEW QUESTIONS

This test is for you and is intended to check your own mastery of the content. Answers are provided in Appendix A.

1. The precordium is:

   a) a synonym for the mediastinum.
   b) the area on the chest where the apical impulse is felt.
   c) the area on the anterior chest overlying the heart and great vessels.
   d) a synonym for the area where the superior and inferior vena cavae return unoxygenated venous blood to the right side of the heart.

2. Select the best description of the tricuspid valve.

   a) left semilunar valve
   b) right atrioventricular valve
   c) left atrioventricular valve
   d) right semilunar valve

3. The function of the pulmonic valve is to:

   a) divide the left atrium and left ventricle.
   b) guard the opening between the right atrium and right ventricle.
   c) protect the orifice between the right ventricle and the pulmonary artery.
   d) guard the entrance to the aorta from the left ventricle.

4. Atrial systole occurs:

   a) during ventricular systole.
   b) during ventricular diastole.
   c) concurrently with ventricular systole.
   d) independently of ventricular function.

5. The second heart sound is the result of:

   a) opening of the mitral and tricuspid valves.
   b) closing of the mitral and tricuspid valves.
   c) opening of the aortic and pulmonic valves.
   d) closing of the aortic and pulmonic valves.

6. The examiner has estimated the jugular venous pressure. Identify the finding that is abnormal.

   a) Patient elevated to 30 degrees, internal jugular vein pulsation at 1 cm above sternal angle.
   b) Patient elevated to 30 degrees, internal jugular vein pulsation at 2 cm above sternal angle.
   c) Patient elevated to 40 degrees, internal jugular vein pulsation at 1 cm above sternal angle.
   d) Patient elevated to 45 degrees, internal jugular vein pulsation at 4 cm above sternal angle.

7. The examiner is palpating the apical impulse. The normal size of this impulse:

   a) is less than 1 cm.
   b) is about 2 cm.
   c) is 3 cm.
   d) varies depending on the size of the person.

8. The examiner wishes to listen in the pulmonic valve area. To do this, the stethoscope would be placed at the:

   a) second right interspace.
   b) second left interspace.
   c) left lower sternal border.
   d) fifth interspace, left midclavicular line.

9. Select the statement that best differentiates a split S_2 from S_3.

   a) S_3 is lower pitched and is heard at the apex.
   b) S_2 is heard at the left lower sternal border.
   c) The timing of S_2 varies with respirations.
   d) S_3 is heard at the base; timing varies with respirations.

10. The examiner wishes to listen for a pericardial friction rub. Select the best method of listening:

    a) with the diaphragm, patient sitting up and leaning forward, breath held in expiration
    b) using the bell with the patient leaning forward
    c) at the base during normal respiration
    d) with the diaphragm, patient turned to the left side

11. When auscultating the heart, your first step is to:

    a) identify S_1 and S_2.
    b) listen for S_3 and S_4.
    c) listen for murmurs.
    d) identify all four sounds on the first round.

12. You'll hear a split S_2 most clearly in what area?

    a) apical
    b) pulmonic
    c) tricuspid
    d) aortic

13. The stethoscope bell should be pressed lightly against the skin so that:

    a) chest hair doesn't simulate crackles.
    b) high-pitched sounds can be heard better.
    c) it doesn't act as a diaphragm.
    d) it doesn't interfere with amplification of heart sounds.

14. A murmur heard after S_1 and before S_2 is classified as:

    a) diastolic (possibly benign).
    b) diastolic (always pathologic).
    c) systolic (possibly benign).
    d) systolic (always pathologic).

Match column A to column B

Column A

15. _____ tough, fibrous, double-walled sac that surrounds and protects the heart

16. _____ thin layer of endothelial tissue that lines the inner surface of the heart chambers and valves

17. _____ reservoir for holding blood

18. _____ ensures smooth, friction-free movement of the heart muscle

19. _____ muscular pumping chamber

20. _____ muscular wall of the heart

Column B

a. pericardial fluid
b. ventricle
c. endocardium
d. myocardium
e. pericardium
f. atrium

21. Briefly relate the route of a blood cell from the liver to tissue in the body.

22. List the major risk factors of heart disease and stroke identified in the text.

SKILLS LABORATORY/CLINICAL SETTING

You are now ready for the clinical component of the cardiovascular system. The purpose of the clinical component is to practice the regional examination on a peer in the skills laboratory or a patient in the clinical setting and to achieve the following.

CLINICAL OBJECTIVES

1. Demonstrate knowledge of the symptoms related to the cardiovascular system by obtaining a regional health history from a peer or patient.

2. Correctly locate anatomic landmarks on the chest wall of a peer.

3. Using a grease pencil, and with peer's permission, outline borders of the heart, and label auscultatory areas on a peer's chest wall.

4. Demonstrate correct technique for inspection and palpation of the neck vessels.

5. Demonstrate correct techniques for inspection, palpation, and auscultation of the precordium.

6. Record the history and physical examination findings accurately, reach an assessment of the health state, and develop a plan of care.

INSTRUCTIONS

Gather your equipment. Wash your hands. Clean the stethoscope endpiece with an alcohol wipe. Practice the steps of the exam of the cardiovascular system on a peer or on a patient in the clinical area. Record your findings using the regional writeup sheet that follows. The front of the page is intended as a worksheet; the back of the page is intended for your narrative recording using the SOAP format.

NOTES

REGIONAL WRITE-UP—CARDIOVACULAR SYSTEM

Date _____

Patient _____ Age _____ Sex _____ Occupation _____

Examiner _____

I. Health History

	No	Yes, explain
1. Any **chest pain** or tightness?		
2. Any **shortness of breath**?		
3. Use more than one pillow to sleep?		
4. Do you have a **cough**?		
5. Do you seem to **tire easily**?		
6. Facial skin ever turn blue or ashen?		
7. Any **swelling** of feet or legs?		
8. Awaken at night to urinate?		
9. Any past history of heart disease?		
10. Any family history of heart disease?		

11. Assess cardiac risk factors: _____

II. Physical Examination

A. Carotid Arteries

Inspect and palpate

Grade R _____ L _____

(0 = absent, 1+ weak, 2+ normal, 3+ increased, 4+ bounding)

B. Jugular Venous System

External jugular veins (circle one): < collapsed supine
meniscus visible at _____

Internal jugular venous pulsations < not visible
(circle one): visible at _____

C. Precordium

Inspect and palpate

1. Skin color and condition _____
2. Chest wall pulsations _____
3. Heave or lift _____
4. Apical impulse in the _____ at _____

Size _____ Amplitude _____

D. Auscultation

1. Identify anatomic areas where you will listen.
2. Rate and rhythm _____
3. Identify S_1 and S_2 in diagram at right and note any variation:

S_1 S_2 S_1 S_2

S_1 _____

S_2 _____

4. Listen in systole and diastole:
   Extra heart sounds _____
   Systolic murmur _____
   Diastolic murmur _____

REGIONAL WRITE-UP—CARDIOVASCULAR SYSTEM

Summarize your findings using the SOAP format.

Subjective (Reason for seeking care, health history)

Objective (Physical exam findings)   Record findings using diagram

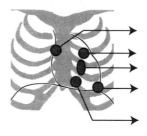

Assessment (Assessment of health state or problem, diagnosis)

Plan (Diagnostic evaluation, follow-up care, patient teaching)

Peripheral Vascular System and Lymphatic System

PURPOSE

This chapter helps you to learn the structure and function of the peripheral vascular system and the lymphatic system; to locate the peripheral pulse sites; to understand the rationale and methods of examination of the peripheral vascular and lymphatic systems; and to accurately record the assessment. At the end of this unit you should be able to perform a complete assessment of the peripheral vascular and lymphatic systems.

READING ASSIGNMENT

Jarvis, *Physical Examination and Health Assessment,* 4th ed., Chapter 20, pp. 533-560.

AUDIO-VISUAL ASSIGNMENT

Jarvis, *Saunders Video Series: Peripheral Vascular System and Lymphatics*

GLOSSARY

Study the following terms after completing the reading assignment. You should be able to cover the definition on the right and define the term out loud.

Allen test....................... determining the patency of the radial and ulnar arteries by compressing one artery site and observing return of skin color as evidence of patency of the other artery

Aneurysm................................ defect or sac formed by dilation in artery wall due to atherosclerosis, trauma, or congenital defect

Arrhythmia .... variation from the heart's normal rhythm

Arteriosclerosis .... thickening and loss of elasticity of the arterial walls

Atherosclerosis........................... plaques of fatty deposits formed in the inner layer (intima) of the arteries

Bradycardia .... slow heart rate, < 50 beats per minute in the adult

Bruit .... blowing, swooshing sound heard through a stethoscope when an artery is partially occluded

Cyanosis .... dusky blue mottling of the skin and mucous membranes due to excessive amount of reduced hemoglobin in the blood

Diastole .... the heart's filling phase

Homans' sign .... calf pain that occurs when the foot is sharply dorsiflexed (pushed up, toward the knee); may occur with deep vein thrombosis, phlebitis, Achilles tendinitis, or muscle injury

Ischemia .... deficiency of arterial blood to a body part, due to constriction or obstruction of a blood vessel

Lymphedema .... swelling of extremity due to obstructed lymph channel, nonpitting

Lymph nodes............................... small oval clumps of lymphatic tissue located at grouped intervals along lymphatic vessels

Pitting edema .... indentation left after examiner depresses the skin over swollen edematous tissue

Profile sign .... viewing the finger from the side in order to detect early clubbing

Pulse .... pressure wave created by each heartbeat, palpable at body sites where the artery lies close to the skin and over a bone

Pulsus alternans .... regular rhythm, but force of pulse varies with alternating beats of large and small amplitude

Pulsus bigeminus .... irregular rhythm, every other beat is premature; premature beats have weakened amplitude

Pulsus paradoxus .... beats have weaker amplitude with respiratory inspiration, stronger with expiration

Systole.. the heart's pumping phase

Tachycardia .... rapid heart rate, > 100 beats per minute in the adult

Thrombophlebitis .... inflammation of the vein associated with thrombus formation

Varicose vein .... dilated tortuous veins with incompetent valves

Ulcer .... open skin lesion extending into dermis with sloughing of necrotic inflammatory tissue

STUDY GUIDE

After completing the reading assignment and the audio-visual assignment, you should be able to answer the following questions in the spaces provided.

1. Describe the structure and function of arteries and veins.

2. List the pulse sites accessible to examination.

3. Describe 3 mechanisms that help return venous blood to the heart.

4. Define the term *capacitance vessels* and explain its significance.

5. List the risk factors for venous stasis.

6. Describe the function of the lymphatic system.

7. Describe the function of the lymph nodes.

8. Name the related organs in the lymphatic system.

9. List the symptom areas to address during history taking of the peripheral vascular system.

10. Fill in the grading scale for assessing the force of an arterial pulse: 0 = _____; 1+ _____; 2+ _____; 3+ _____; 4+ _____

11. List the steps in performing the modified Allen test.

12. List the skin characteristics expected with arterial insufficiency to the lower legs.

13. Compare the characteristics of leg ulcers associated with arterial insufficiency to ulcers with venous insufficiency.

14. Fill in the description of the grading scale for pitting edema:

1+ _____

2+ _____

3+ _____

4+ _____

15. Describe the technique for using the Doppler ultrasonic stethoscope to detect peripheral pulses.

16. Raynaud's phenomenon has associated progressive tricolor changes of the skin from _____ to _____ and then to _____. State the mechanism for each of these color changes.

ASSESSMENT VIDEO CRITICAL THINKING QUESTIONS

Discussion answers to these questions are in the Instructor's Manual for *Physical Examination and Health Assessment*, 4th ed.

1. Which assessment findings are you likely to see in a patient who seeks care because of leg pain or cramps?

2. How do ulcers caused by chronic arterial insufficiency compare to those of chronic venous insufficiency?

3. How may aging affect your findings when examining an older adult's peripheral vascular and lymphatic systems?

4. What nursing diagnoses commonly are related to abnormal findings in the peripheral vascular system?

Fill in the labels indicated on the following arteries and pulse sites.

REVIEW QUESTIONS

This test is for you and is intended to check your own mastery of the content. Answers are provided in Appendix A.

1. A function of the venous system is:

    a) to hold more blood when blood volume increases.
    b) to conserve fluid and plasma proteins that leak out of the capillaries.
    c) to form a major part of the immune system that defends the body against disease.
    d) to absorb lipids from the intestinal tract.

2. The organs that aid the lymphatic system are:

    a) liver, lymph nodes, and stomach.
    b) pancreas, small intestines, and thymus.
    c) spleen, tonsils, and thymus.
    d) pancreas, spleen, and tonsils.

3. Ms. T. has come for a prenatal visit. She complains of dependent edema, varicosities in the legs, and hemorrhoids. The best response is:

    a) "If these symptoms persist, we will perform an amniocentesis."
    b) "If these symptoms persist, we will discuss having you hospitalized."
    c) "The symptoms are caused by the pressure of the growing uterus on the veins. They are usual conditions of pregnancy."
    d) "At this time, the symptoms are a minor inconvenience. You should learn to accept them."

4. A pulse with an amplitude of 3+ would be considered:

    a) bounding.
    b) increased.
    c) normal.
    d) weak.

5. Inspection of a person's right hand reveals a red, swollen area. To further assess for infection, you would palpate the:

    a) cervical node.
    b) axillary node.
    c) epitrochlear node.
    d) inguinal node.

6. In order to screen for deep vein thrombosis, you would:

    a) measure the circumference of the ankle.
    b) check the temperature with the palm of the hand.
    c) compress the dorsalis pedis pulse, looking for blood return.
    d) measure the widest point with a tape measure.

7. During the examination of the lower extremities, you are unable to palpate the popliteal pulse. You should:

    a) proceed with the exam. It is often impossible to palpate this pulse.
    b) refer the patient to a vascular surgeon for further evaluation.
    c) schedule the patient for a venogram.
    d) schedule the patient for an arteriogram.

8. While reviewing a medical record, a notation of 4+ edema of the right leg is noted. The best description of this type of edema is:

    a) mild pitting, no perceptible swelling of the leg.
    b) moderate pitting, indentation subsides rapidly.
    c) deep pitting, leg looks swollen.
    d) very deep pitting, indentation lasts a long time.

9. The examiner wishes to assess for arterial deficit in the lower extremities. After raising the legs 12 inches off the table and then having the person sit up and dangle the leg, the color should return in:

   a) 5 seconds or less.
   b) 10 seconds or less.
   c) 15 seconds.
   d) 30 seconds.

10. A 54-year-old woman with five children has varicose veins of the lower extremities. Her most characteristic sign is:

    a) reduced arterial circulation.
    b) blanching, deathlike appearance of the extremities on elevation.
    c) loss of hair on feet and toes.
    d) dilated, tortuous superficial bluish vessels.

11. Atrophic skin changes that occur with peripheral arterial insufficiency include:

    a) thin, shiny skin with loss of hair.
    b) brown discoloration.
    c) thick, leathery skin.
    d) slow-healing blisters on the skin.

12. Intermittent claudication is:

    a) muscular pain relieved by exercise.
    b) neurologic pain relieved by exercise.
    c) muscular pain brought on by exercise.
    d) neurologic pain brought on by exercise.

13. A known risk factor for venous ulcer development is:

    a) obesity.
    b) male gender.
    c) history of hypertension.
    d) daily aspirin therapy.

14. Brawny edema is:

    a) acute in onset.
    b) soft.
    c) nonpitting.
    d) associated with diminished pulses.

SKILLS LABORATORY/CLINICAL SETTING

You are now ready for the clinical component of the peripheral vascular system. The purpose of the clinical component is to practice the regional examination on a peer in the skills laboratory or a patient in the clinical setting and to achieve the following.

CLINICAL OBJECTIVES

1. Demonstrate knowledge of the symptoms related to the peripheral vascular system by obtaining a regional health history from a peer or patient.

2. Demonstrate palpation of peripheral arterial pulses (brachial, radial, femoral, popliteal, posterior tibial, dorsalis pedis) by: assessing amplitude and symmetry; noting any signs of arterial insufficiency.

3. Demonstrate inspection and palpation of peripheral veins by noting any signs of venous insufficiency.

4. Demonstrate palpation of lymphatic system by identifying enlargement, clumping, or abnormal firmness of regional lymph nodes.

5. Demonstrate correct technique for performing the following additional tests when indicated: Allen test; Trendelenburg's test; manual compression test; Doppler ultrasonic stethoscope; computing the ankle-arm index.

6. Record the history and physical examination findings accurately, reach an assessment of the health state, and develop a plan of care.

INSTRUCTIONS

Gather your equipment. Wash your hands. Practice the steps of the exam of the peripheral vascular system on a peer or on a patient in the clinical setting, giving appropriate instructions as you proceed. Record your findings using the regional write-up sheets that follow. The first part is intended as a worksheet; the last page is intended for your narrative summary recording using the SOAP format. Note that the peripheral examination and cardiovascular examination usually are practiced together.

NOTES

REGIONAL WRITE-UP—PERIPHERAL VASCULAR SYSTEM   Date _____

Patient _____ Age _____ Sex _____ Occupation _____

Examiner _____

I. Health History

	No	Yes, explain
1. Any leg **pain** (cramps)? Where?		
2. Any **skin changes** in arms or legs?		
3. Any sores or **lesions** in arms or legs?		
4. Any **swelling** in the legs?		
5. Any **swollen glands**? Where?		
6. What medications are you taking?		

II. Physical Examination

A. Inspection

1. The Arms

Inspect

Color of skin and nailbeds _____

Symmetry _____

Lesions _____

Edema _____

Clubbing _____

Palpate _____

Temperature _____

Texture _____

Capillary refill _____

Locate and grade pulses (record on back)

Check epitrochlear lymph node _____

Modified Allen test (if indicated) _____

2. The Legs

Inspect

Color _____

Hair distribution _____

Venous pattern/varicosities _____

Size _____

Swelling/edema _____

Atrophy _____

If so, measure calf circumference in cm R _____ L _____

Skin lesions or ulcers _____

Palpate

Temperature _____

Check Homans' sign _____

Tenderness _____

Inguinal lymph nodes _____

Locate and grade pulses (record on back)

Check pretibial edema (grade if present) _____

Auscultate for bruit (if indicated) _____

REGIONAL WRITE-UP—PERIPHERAL VASCULAR SYSTEM

	Brachial	Radial	Femoral	Popliteal	D. pedis	P. tibial
R						
L						

0 = absent; 1+ weak; 2+ normal; 3+ full; 4+ bounding

3. Additional Tests
   Manual compression test _____
   Trendelenburg's test _____
   Check color change: elevate legs, then dangle; color returns in _____ seconds
   Doppler ultrasonic stethoscope
      Locate pulse sites
      Ankle-brachial index (ABI)
      _____ankle systolic pressure
      _____ = _____. _____ or _____%
      _____ arm systolic pressure

REGIONAL WRITE-UP—PERIPHERAL VASCULAR SYSTEM

Summarize your findings using the SOAP format.

Subjective (Reason for seeking care, health history)

Objective (Physical exam findings) (Record pulses on diagram below)

Assessment (Assessment of health state or problem, diagnosis)

Plan (Diagnostic evaluation, follow-up care, teaching)

CHAPTER 21

Abdomen

GLOSSARY

Study the following terms after completing the reading assignment. You should be able to cover the definition on the right and define the term out loud.

Aneurysm... defect or sac formed by dilation in artery wall due to atherosclerosis, trauma, or congenital defect

Anorexia .... loss of appetite for food

Ascites... abnormal accumulation of serous fluid within the peritoneal cavity, associated with congestive heart failure, cirrhosis, cancer, or portal hypertension

Borborygmi .... loud gurgling bowel sounds signaling increased motility or hyperperistalsis, occur with early bowel obstruction, gastroenteritis, diarrhea

Bruit... blowing, swooshing sound heard through a stethoscope when an artery is partially occluded

Cecum... first or proximal part of large intestine

Cholecystitis .... inflammation of the gallbladder

Costal margin .... lower border of rib margin formed by the medial edges of the 8th, 9th, and 10th ribs

Costovertebral angle (CVA) ...... angle formed by the 12th rib and the vertebral column on the posterior thorax, overlying the kidney

Diastasis recti .... midline longitudinal ridge in the abdomen, a separation of abdominal rectus muscles

Dysphagia .... difficulty swallowing

Epigastrium .... name of abdominal region between the costal margins

Hepatomegaly .... abnormal enlargement of liver

Hernia .... abnormal protrusion of bowel through weakening in abdominal musculature

Inguinal ligament .... ligament extending from pubic bone to anterior superior iliac spine, forming lower border of abdomen

Linea alba .... midline tendinous seam joining the abdominal muscles

Paralytic ileus .... complete absence of peristaltic movement that may follow abdominal surgery or complete bowel obstruction

Peritoneal friction rub .... rough grating sound heard through the stethoscope over the site of peritoneal inflammation

Peritonitis .... inflammation of peritoneum

Pyloric stenosis .... congenital narrowing of pyloric sphincter, forming outflow obstruction of stomach

Pyrosis .... (heartburn) burning sensation in upper abdomen, due to reflux of gastric acid

Rectus abdominis muscle .... midline abdominal muscles extending from rib cage to pubic bone

Scaphoid .... abnormally sunken abdominal wall as with malnutrition or underweight

Splenomegaly .... abnormal enlargement of spleen

Striae .... (linea albicantes) silvery white or pink scar tissue formed by stretching of abdominal skin as with pregnancy or obesity

Suprapubic .... name of abdominal region just superior to pubic bone

Tympany .... high-pitched, musical, drumlike percussion note heard when percussing over the stomach and intestine

Umbilicus .... depression on the abdomen marking site of entry of umbilical cord

Viscera .... internal organs

STUDY GUIDE

After completing the reading assignment and the audio-visual assignment, you should be able to answer the following questions in the spaces provided.

1. Draw a picture of the abdomen and label its contents.

2. Name the organs that are normally palpable in the abdomen.

3. Describe the proper positioning and preparation of the patient for the exam.

4. State the rationale for performing auscultation of the abdomen before palpation or percussion.

5. Discuss inspection of the abdomen, including findings that should be noted.

6. Describe the procedure for auscultation of bowel sounds.

7. Differentiate the following abdominal sounds: normal, hyperactive, and hypoactive bowel sounds, succession splash, bruit.

8. Identify and give the rationale for each of the percussion notes heard over the abdomen.

List 4 conditions that may alter normal percussion notes.

9. Describe the procedure for percussing the liver span and the spleen.

10. Describe these maneuvers and discuss their significance: fluid wave test, shifting dullness.

11. Differentiate between light and deep palpation, and explain the purpose of each.

List 2 abnormalities that may be detected by light palpation and 2 detected by deep palpation.

12. Contrast rigidity with voluntary guarding.

13. Contrast visceral pain and somatic (parietal) pain.

14. Describe rebound tenderness.

15. Describe palpation of the liver, spleen, kidney.

16. Distinguish abdominal wall masses from intra-abdominal masses.

17. Describe the procedure and rationale for determining costovertebral angle (CVA) tenderness.

18. Describe the expected examination findings of the abdomen in each of the following conditions:

Obesity _____

Gaseous distention _____

Tumor _____

Pregnancy _____

Ascites _____

Enlarged liver _____

Enlarged spleen _____

Distended bladder _____

Appendicitis _____

ASSESSMENT VIDEO CRITICAL THINKING QUESTIONS

Discussion answers to these questions are in the Instructor's Manual for *Physical Examination and Health Assessment*, 4th ed.

1. Describe common sites of referred abdominal pain.

2. What bowel sounds would you expect to hear in a patient with diarrhea?

3. What abnormal findings can be detected by light palpation of the abdomen?

4. What should you suspect if your palpation detects an enlarged spleen? What should you do next?

Fill in the labels indicated on the following illustrations.

REVIEW QUESTIONS

This test is for you and is intended to check your own mastery of the content. Answers are provided in Appendix A.

1. Select the sequence of techniques used during an examination of the abdomen.

   a) percussion, inspection, palpation, auscultation
   b) inspection, palpation, percussion, auscultation
   c) inspection, auscultation, percussion, palpation
   d) auscultation, inspection, palpation, percussion

2. Which of the following may be noted through inspection of the abdomen?

   a) fluid waves and abdominal contour
   b) umbilical eversion and Murphy's sign
   c) venous pattern, peristaltic waves, and abdominal contour
   d) peritoneal irritation, general tympany, and peristaltic waves

3. Right upper quadrant tenderness may indicate pathology in the:

   a) liver, pancreas, or ascending colon.
   b) liver and stomach.
   c) sigmoid colon, spleen, or rectum.
   d) appendix or ileocecal valve.

4. Hyperactive bowel sounds are:

   a) high pitched.
   b) rushing.
   c) tinkling.
   d) all of the above.

5. The absence of bowel sounds is established after listening for:

   a) 1 full minute.
   b) 3 full minutes.
   c) 5 full minutes.
   d) none of the above.

6. Auscultation of the abdomen may reveal bruits of the _____ arteries.

   a) aortic, renal, iliac, and femoral
   b) jugular, aortic, carotid, and femoral
   c) pulmonic, aortic, and portal
   d) renal, iliac, internal jugular, and basilic

7. The range of normal liver span in the right mid-clavicular line in the adult is:

   a) 2–6 cm.
   b) 4–8 cm.
   c) 8–14 cm.
   d) 6–12 cm.

8. The left upper quadrant (LUQ) contains the:

   a) liver.
   b) appendix.
   c) left ovary.
   d) spleen.

9. Striae, which occur when the elastic fibers in the reticular layer of the skin are broken following rapid or prolonged stretching, have a distinct color when of long duration. This color is:

   a) pink.
   b) blue.
   c) purple-blue.
   d) silvery white.

10. Auscultation of the abdomen is begun in the right lower quadrant (RLQ) because:

    a) bowel sounds are always normally present here.
    b) peristalsis through the descending colon is usually active.
    c) this is the location of the pyloric sphincter.
    d) vascular sounds are best heard in this area.

11. A dull percussion note forward of the left midaxillary line is:

    a) normal, an expected finding during splenic percussion.
    b) expected between the 8th and 12th ribs.
    c) found if the exam follows a large meal.
    d) indicative of splenic enlargement.

12. Shifting dullness is a test for:

    a) ascites.
    b) splenic enlargement.
    c) inflammation of the kidney.
    d) hepatomegaly.

13. Tenderness during abdominal palpation is expected when palpating:

    a) the liver edge.
    b) the spleen.
    c) the sigmoid colon.
    d) the kidneys.

14. Murphy's sign is best described as:

    a) the pain felt when the hand of the examiner is rapidly removed from an inflamed appendix.
    b) pain felt when taking a deep breath when the examiner's fingers are on the approximate location of the inflamed gallbladder.
    c) a sharp pain felt by the patient when one hand of the examiner is used to thump the other at the costovertebral angle.
    d) not a valid examination technique.

SKILLS LABORATORY/CLINICAL SETTING

You are now ready for the clinical component of the abdominal system. The purpose of the clinical component is to practice the regional examination on a peer in the skills laboratory or a patient in the clinical setting and to achieve the following.

CLINICAL OBJECTIVES

1. Demonstrate knowledge of the symptoms related to the abdominal system by obtaining a regional health history from a peer or patient.

2. Demonstrate inspection of the abdomen by assessing skin condition, symmetry, contour, pulsation, umbilicus, nutritional state.

3. Demonstrate auscultation of the abdomen by assessing characteristics of bowel sounds and by screening for bruits.

4. Demonstrate percussion of the abdomen by: identifying predominant percussion note; determining liver span; noting borders of spleen.

5. Demonstrate light palpation by assessing muscular resistance, tenderness, any masses.

6. Demonstrate deep palpation by assessing for: any masses; the liver, spleen, kidneys, aorta; any CVA or rebound tenderness.

7. Demonstrate correct technique of performing the following additional tests when indicated: inspiratory arrest; iliopsoas muscle test; obturator test.

8. Record the history and physical examination findings accurately, reach an assessment of the health state, and develop a plan of care.

INSTRUCTIONS

Gather your equipment. Wash your hands. Assess the patient's comfort before starting. Practice the steps of the exam on a peer or a patient in the clinical setting, giving appropriate instructions as you proceed. Record your findings using the regional write-up sheets that follow. The front of the page is intended as a worksheet; the back of the page is intended for your narrative summary recording using the SOAP format.

NOTES

REGIONAL WRITE-UP—ABDOMEN EXAMINAITON   Date _____

Patient _____ Age _____ Sex _____ Occupation _____

Examiner _____

I. Health History

	No	Yes, explain

1. Any change in **appetite**? Loss? _____
2. Any difficulty **swallowing**? _____
3. Any foods you **cannot tolerate**? _____
4. Any **abdominal pain**? _____
5. Any **nausea** or **vomiting**? _____
6. How often are **bowel movements**? _____
7. Any past history of **GI disease**? _____
8. What **medications** are you taking? _____
9. Tell me all food you ate in the last **24 hours**, starting with:

    breakfast   snack   lunch   snack   dinner   snack

II. Physical Examination

A. Inspection

Contour of abdomen _____

General symmetry _____

Skin color and condition _____

Pulsation or movement _____

Umbilicus _____

Hair distribution _____

State of hydration and nutrition _____

Person's facial expression and position in bed _____

B. Auscultation

Bowel sounds _____

Note any vascular sounds _____

C. Percussion

Percuss in all four quadrants _____

Percuss borders of liver span in R MCL _____cm _____

Percuss spleen _____

If suspect ascites, test for fluid wave and shifting dullness _____

D. Palpation

Light palpation in all four quadrants

    Muscle wall _____

    Tenderness _____

    Enlarged organs _____

    Masses _____

Deep palpation in all four quadrants _____

    Masses _____

    Contour of liver _____

    Spleen _____

    Kidneys _____

Aorta _____

Rebound tenderness _____

CVA tenderness _____

E. Additional tests, if indicated

REGIONAL WRITE-UP—ABDOMEN

Summarize your findings using the SOAP format.

Subjective (Reason for seeking care, health history)

Objective (Physical exam findings)

Record findings on diagram.

Assessment (Assessment of health state or problem, diagnosis)

Plan (Diagnostic evaluation, follow-up care, patient teaching)

CHAPTER 22

Musculoskeletal System

PURPOSE

This chapter helps you to learn the structure and function of the various joints in the body; to know their normal ranges of motion; to position the patient comfortably during the examination; to understand the rationale and methods of examination of the musculoskeletal system; to assess functional ability; and to accurately record the assessment. At the end of this unit you should be able to perform a complete assessment of the musculoskeletal system.

READING ASSIGNMENT

Jarvis, *Physical Examination and Health Assessment*, 4th ed., Chapter 22, pp. 601-660.

AUDIO-VISUAL ASSIGNMENT

Jarvis, *Saunders Video Series: Musculoskeletal System*

GLOSSARY

Study the following terms after completing the reading assignment. You should be able to cover the definition on the right and define the term out loud.

Abduction .... moving a body part away from an axis or the median line

Adduction .... moving a body part toward the center or toward the median line

Ankylosis .... immobility, consolidation, and fixation of a joint because of disease, injury, or surgery; most often due to chronic rheumatoid arthritis

Ataxia .... inability to perform coordinated movements

Bursa .... enclosed sac filled with viscous fluid located in joint areas of potential friction

Circumduction .... moving the arm in a circle around the shoulder

Crepitation .... dry crackling sound or sensation due to grating of the ends of damaged bone

Dorsa .... directed toward or located on the surface

Dupuytren's contracture .... flexion contractures of the fingers due to chronic hyperplasia of the palmar fascia

Eversion .... moving the sole of the foot outward at the ankle

Extension .... straightening a limb at a joint

Flexion .... bending a limb at a joint

Ganglion .... round, cystic, nontender nodule overlying a tendon sheath or joint capsule, usually on dorsum of wrist

Hallux valgus .... lateral or outward deviation of the great toe

Inversion .... moving the sole of the foot inward at the ankle

Kyphosis .... outward or convex curvature of the thoracic spine, hunchback

Ligament .... fibrous bands running directly from one bone to another bone that strengthen the joint

Lordosis .... inward or concave curvature of the lumbar spine

Nucleus pulposus .... center of the intervertebral disc

Olecranon process .... bony projection of the ulna at the elbow

Patella .... kneecap

Plantar .... surface of the sole of the foot

Pronation .... turning the forearm so that the palm is down

Protraction .... moving a body part forward and parallel to the ground

Range of motion (ROM) .... extent of movement of a joint

Retraction .... moving a body part backward and parallel to the ground

Rheumatoid arthritis .... chronic systemic inflammatory disease of joints and surrounding connective tissue

Sciatica .... nerve pain along the course of the sciatic nerve that travels down from the back or thigh through the leg and into the foot

Scoliosis .... S-shaped curvature of the thoracic spine

Supination .... turning the forearm so that the palm is up

Talipes equinovarus .... (clubfoot) congenital deformity of the foot in which it is plantar flexed and inverted

Tendon .... strong fibrous cord that attaches a skeletal muscle to a bone

Torticollis .... (wryneck) contraction of the cervical neck muscles, producing torsion of the neck

STUDY GUIDE

After completing the reading assignment and the audio-visual assignment, you should be able to answer the following questions in the spaces provided.

1. List 4 signs that suggest acute inflammation in a joint.

2. Differentiate the following:

   dislocation

   subluxation

   contracture

   ankylosis

3. Describe the correct method for use of the goniometer.

4. Differentiate testing of active range of motion versus passive range of motion.

5. State the expected range of degrees of flexion and extension of the following joints:

   elbow

   wrist

   fingers (at metacarpophalangeal joints)

6. State the expected range of degrees of flexion and extension of the following joints:

   hip

   knee

   ankle

7. Explain the method for measuring leg length.

8. Describe the Ortolani maneuver for checking an infant's hips.

9. State 4 landmarks to note when checking an adolescent for scoliosis.

10. When performing a functional assessment for an older adult, state the common adaptations the aging person makes when attempting these maneuvers:

Walking _____

Climbing up stairs _____

Walking down stairs _____

Picking up object from floor _____

Rising up from sitting in chair _____

Rising up from lying in bed _____

11. Describe the symptoms and signs in carpal tunnel syndrome.

Name and describe 2 techniques of examination for the syndrome.

12. Draw and describe swan neck deformity and boutonniere deformity.

13. Contrast Bouchard's nodes from Heberden's nodes.

14. Contrast syndactyly and polydactyly.

ASSESSMENT VIDEO CRITICAL THINKING QUESTIONS

Discussion answers to these questions are in the Instructor's Manual for *Physical Examination and Health Assessment*, 4th ed.

1. What other assessment findings can you expect to see in a patient who reports joint pain?

2. What abnormal findings may commonly be detected during assessment of the wrists and hands?

3. When are genu varum and genu valgum considered normal? What abnormal conditions may also cause them?

4. How does musculoskeletal assessment of an adolescent differ from that of an adult?

Fill in the labels indicated on the following illustrations.

REVIEW QUESTIONS

This test is for you and is intended to check your own mastery of the content. Answers are provided in Appendix A.

1. During an assessment of the spine, the patient would be asked to:

   a) adduct and extend.
   b) supinate, evert, and retract.
   c) extend, adduct, invert, and rotate.
   d) flex, extend, abduct, and rotate.

2. Pronation and supination of the hand and forearm are the result of the articulation of the:

   a) scapula and clavicle.
   b) radius and ulna.
   c) patella and condyle of fibula.
   d) femur and acetabulum.

3. Anterior and posterior stability is provided to the knee joint by the:

   a) medial and lateral menisci.
   b) patellar tendon and ligament.
   c) medial collateral ligament and quadriceps muscle.
   d) anterior and posterior cruciate ligaments.

4. A 70-year-old woman has come for a health exam. Which of the following is a common age-related change in the curvature of the spinal column?

   a) lordosis
   b) scoliosis
   c) kyphosis
   d) lateral scoliosis

5. The timing of joint pain may assist the examiner in determining the cause. The joint pain associated with rheumatic fever would:

   a) be worse in the morning.
   b) be worse later in the day.
   c) be worse in the morning but improve during the day.
   d) occur 10 to 14 days after an untreated sore throat.

6. Examination of the shoulder includes four motions. These are:

   a) forward flexion, internal rotation, abduction, and external rotation.
   b) abduction, adduction, pronation, and supination.
   c) circumduction, inversion, eversion, and rotation.
   d) elevation, retraction, protraction, and circumduction.

7. The bulge sign is a test for:

   a) swelling in the suprapatellar pouch.
   b) carpal tunnel syndrome.
   c) Heberden's nodes.
   d) olecranon bursa inflammation.

8. The examiner is going to measure the patient's legs for length discrepancy. The normal finding would be:

   a) no difference in measurements.
   b) 0.5 cm difference.
   c) within 1 cm of each other.
   d) 2 cm difference.

9. A 2-year-old child has been brought to the clinic for a health examination. A common finding would be:

   a) kyphosis.
   b) lordosis.
   c) scoliosis.
   d) no deviation is normal.

10. Briefly describe the functions of the musculoskeletal system.

Match column A with column B.

Column A—Movement

11. _____ Flexion

12. _____ Extension

13. _____ Abduction

14. _____ Adduction

15. _____ Pronation

16. _____ Supination

17. _____ Circumduction

18. _____ Inversion

19. _____ Eversion

20. _____ Rotation

21. _____ Protraction

22. _____ Retraction

23. _____ Elevation

24. _____ Depression

Column B—Description

a. turning the forearm so that the palm is up

b. bending a limb at a joint

c. lowering a body part

d. turning the forearm so that the palm is down

e. straightening a limb at a joint

f. raising a body part

g. moving a limb away from the midline of the body

h. moving a body part backward and parallel to the ground

i. moving a limb toward the midline of the body

j. moving the arm in a circle around the shoulder

k. moving the sole of the foot outward at the ankle

l. moving a body part forward and parallel to the ground

m. moving the sole of the foot inward at the ankle

n. moving the head around a central axis

SKILLS LABORATORY/CLINICAL SETTING

You are now ready for the clinical component of the musculoskeletal system. The purpose of the clinical component is to practice the regional examination on a peer in the skills laboratory or a patient in the clinical setting and to achieve the following.

CLINICAL OBJECTIVES

1. Demonstrate knowledge of the symptoms related to the musculoskeletal system by obtaining a regional health history from a peer or patient.

2. Demonstrate inspection and palpation of the musculoskeletal system by assessing the muscles, bones, and joints for size, symmetry, swelling, nodules, deformities, atrophy, and active range of motion.

3. Assess the person's ability to carry out functional activities of daily living.

4. Record the history and physical examination findings accurately, reach an assessment about the health state, and develop a plan of care.

INSTRUCTIONS

Gather your equipment. Wash your hands. Practice the steps of the exam on a peer or a patient in the clinical setting, giving appropriate instructions as you proceed, and maintaining the safety of the person during movement. Record your findings using the regional write-up sheet that follows. The first section is intended as a worksheet; the last page is intended for your narrative summary recording using the SOAP format.

Note the student performance checklist that follows the regional write-up sheet. It lists the essential behaviors you should display as an examiner, and it may be used by your clinical instructor to evaluate your clinical musculoskeletal examination.

NOTES

REGIONAL WRITE-UP—MUSCULOSKELETAL SYSTEM

Date _____

Patient _____ Age _____ Sex _____ Occupation _____

Examiner _____

I. Health History

	No	Yes, explain
1. Any **pain** in the joints?		
2. Any **stiffness** in the joints?		
3. Any **swelling, heat, redness** in joints?		
4. Any **limitation of movement**?		
5. Any **muscle pain** or cramping?		
6. Any **deformity** of bone or joint?		
7. Any **accidents or trauma** to bones?		
8. Ever had **back pain**?		
9. Any problems with the activities of daily living: bathing, toileting, dressing, grooming, eating, mobility, communicating?		

II. Physical Examination

A. Cervical Spine

1. Inspect size and contour
   Color, swelling
   Mass or deformity
2. Palpate for temperature
   Pain
   Swelling or mass
3. Active range of motion
   Flexion _____ extension _____
   Lateral bending right _____ left _____
   Right rotation _____ left _____

B. Shoulders

1. Inspect size and contour
   Color, swelling
   Mass or deformity
2. Palpate for temperature
   Pain
   Swelling or mass
3. Active range of motion
   Flexion _____ extension _____
   Abduction _____ adduction _____
   Internal rotation _____ external rotation _____

C. Elbows

1. Inspect for size and contour
   Color, swelling
   Mass or deformity
2. Palpate for temperature
   Pain
   Swelling or mass
3. Active range of motion
   Flexion _____ extension _____
   Pronation _____ supination _____

D. Wrists and hands

1. Inspect for size and contour
   Color, swelling
   Mass or deformity
2. Palpate for temperature
   Pain
   Swelling or mass
3. Active range of motion
   Wrist extension _____ flexion _____
   Finger extension_____ flexion _____
   Ulnar deviation_____ radial deviation _____
   Fingers spread_____ make fist _____
   Touch thumb to each finger _____

E. Hips

1. Inspect size and contour
   Color, swelling
   Mass or deformity
2. Palpate for temperature
   Pain
   Swelling or mass
3. Active range of motion
   Extension _____ flexion _____
   External rotation _____ internal rotation _____
   Abduction _____ adduction _____

F. Knees

1. Inspect size and contour
   Color, swelling
   Mass or deformity
2. Palpate for temperature
   Pain
   Swelling or mass
3. Active range of motion
   Flexion _____ extension _____
   Walk _____ shallow knee bend _____

G. Ankles and feet
   1. Inspect for size and contour
      Color, swelling
      Mass or deformity
   2. Palpate for temperature
      Pain
      Swelling or mass
   3. Active range of motion
      Dorsiflexion _____ plantar flexion _____
      Inversion _____ eversion _____

H. Spine
   1. Inspect for straight spinous processes
      Equal horizontal positions for: shoulders, scapulae, iliac crests, gluteal folds
      Equal spaces between arms and lateral thorax
      Knees and feet align with trunk, point forward
      From side note curvature: cervical, thoracic, lumbar
   2. Palpate spinous processes
   3. Active range of motion
      Flexion _____ extension _____
      Lateral bending right _____ left _____
      Rotation right _____ left _____

I. Additional tests (if indicated)
   Phalen's test
   Tinel's sign
   Bulge sign
   Ballottement
   McMurray's test
   Straight leg raising
   Measure leg-length discrepancy

J. Functional assessment (if indicated)
   Walk (with shoes on)
   Climb up stairs
   Walk down stairs
   Pick up object from floor
   Rise up from sitting in chair
   Rise up from lying in bed

REGONAL WRITE-UP—MUSCULOSKELETAL SYSTEM

Summarize your findings using the SOAP format.

Subjective (Reason for seeking care, health history)

Objective (Physical exam findings)

Assessment (Assessment of health state or problem, diagnosis)

Plan (Diagnostic evaluation, follow-up care, patient teaching)

STUDENT PERFORMANCE CHECKLIST

MUSCULOSKELETAL SYSTEM—Essential Behaviors

	Yes	No	Comments
Obtain relevant history, functional and self-care assessments			
Gather equipment			
tape measure			
goniometer			
skin marking pen			
light if needed			
Provide privacy			
Wash hands			
Observe for symmetry			
Inspect each joint for: size			
contour			
range of motion/limitation			
Inspect skin and tissue over joints for: color			
swelling			
masses			
deformity			
Palpate each joint for: heat			
tenderness			
swelling			
masses			
Test ROM			
Grade muscle strength			
Record findings including notations regarding specific joints			
temporomandibular			
cervical spine			

	Yes	No	Comments
shoulders			
elbow			
wrist			
hand			
hip			
knee			
Ballottement test			
McMurray's test			
ankle			
foot			
Document findings			

CHAPTER

Neurologic System

PURPOSE

This chapter helps you to learn the structure and function of the components of the neurologic system including the cranial nerves, cerebellar system, motor system, sensory system, and reflexes; to understand the rationale and methods of examination of the neurologic system; and to accurately record the assessment. Together with the mental status assessment presented in Chapter 6, you should be able to perform a complete assessment of the neurologic system, at the end of this unit.

READING ASSIGNMENT

Jarvis, *Physical Examination and Health Assessment*, 4th ed., Chapter 23 pp. 661-720.

AUDIO-VISUAL ASSIGNMENT

Jarvis, *Saunders Video Series, Physical Examination and Health Assessment: Neurologic: Cranial Nerves and Sensory System; Neurologic: Motor System and Reflexes*

GLOSSARY

Study the following terms after completing the reading assignment. You should be able to cover the definition on the right and define the term out loud.

Agnosia..................................... loss of ability to recognize importance of sensory impressions

Agraphia.................................... loss of ability to express thoughts in writing

Amnesia..................................... loss of memory

Analgesia................................... loss of pain sensation

Aphasia...................................... loss of power of expression by speech, writing, or signs, or of comprehension of spoken or written language

Apraxia...................................... loss of ability to perform purposeful movements in the absence of sensory or motor damage, e.g., inability to use objects correctly

Ataxia .... inability to perform coordinated movements

Athetosis .... bizarre, slow, twisting, writhing movement, resembling a snake or worm

Chorea .... sudden, rapid, jerky, purposeless movement involving limbs, trunk, or face

Clonus .... rapidly alternating involuntary contraction and relaxation of a muscle in response to sudden stretch

Coma .... state of profound unconsciousness from which person cannot be aroused

Decerebrate rigidity .... arms stiffly extended, adducted, internally rotated; legs stiffly extended, plantar flexed

Decorticate rigidity .... arms adducted and flexed, wrists and fingers flexed; legs extended, internally rotated, plantar flexed

Dysarthria .... imperfect articulation of speech due to problems of muscular control resulting from central or peripheral nervous system damage

Dysphasia .... impairment in speech consisting of lack of coordination and inability to arrange words in their proper order

Extinction .... disappearance of conditioned response

Fasciculation .... rapid continuous twitching of resting muscle without movement of limb

Flaccidity .... loss of muscle tone, limp

Graphesthesia .... ability to "read" a number by having it traced on the skin

Hemiplegia .... loss of motor power (paralysis) on one side of the body, usually caused by a cerebral vascular accident; paralysis occurs on the side opposite the lesion

Lower motor neuron .... motor neuron in the peripheral nervous system with its nerve fiber extending out to the muscle and only its cell body in the central nervous system

Myoclonus .... rapid sudden jerk of a muscle

Nuchal rigidity .... stiffness in cervical neck area

Nystagmus .... back-and-forth oscillation of the eyes

Opisthotonos .... prolonged arching of back, with head and heels bent backward, and meningeal irritation

Paralysis .... decreased or loss of motor function due to problem with motor nerve or muscle fibers

Paraplegia .... impairment or loss of motor and/or sensory function in the lower half of the body

Paresthesia .... abnormal sensation, i.e., burning, numbness, tingling, prickling, crawling skin sensation

Point localization .... ability of the person to discriminate exactly where on the body the skin has been touched

Proprioception .... sensory information concerning body movements and position of the body in space

Spasticity .... continuous resistance to stretching by a muscle due to abnormally increased tension, with increased deep tendon reflexes

Stereognosis .... ability to recognize objects by feeling their forms, sizes, and weights while the eyes are closed

Tic .... repetitive twitching of a muscle group at inappropriate times, e.g., wink, grimace

Tremor .... involuntary contraction of opposing muscle groups resulting in rhythmic movement of one or more joints

Two-point discrimination .... ability to distinguish the separation of two simultaneous pin pricks on the skin

Upper motor neuron .... nerve located entirely within the central nervous system

STUDY GUIDE

After completing the reading assignment and the audio-visual assignment, you should be able to answer the following questions in the spaces provided.

1. List the major function(s) of the following components of the central nervous system:

   Cerebral cortex—frontal lobe _____

   Cerebral cortex—parietal lobe _____

   Cerebral cortex—temporal lobe _____

   Cerebral cortex—Wernicke's area _____

   Cerebral cortex—Broca's area _____

   Basal ganglia _____

   Thalamus _____

   Hypothalamus _____

   Cerebellum _____

   Midbrain _____

   Pons _____

   Medulla _____

   Spinal cord _____

2. List the primary sensations mediated by the two major sensory pathways of the CNS.

3. Describe 3 major motor pathways in the CNS including the type of movements mediated by each.

4. Differentiate an upper motor neuron from a lower motor neuron.

5. List the 5 components of a deep tendon reflex arc.

6. List the major symptom areas to assess when collecting a health history for the neurologic system.

7. List the method of testing for each of the 12 cranial nerves.

8. List and describe 3 tests of cerebellar function.

9. Describe the method of testing the sensory system for pain, temperature, touch, vibration, and position.

10. Define the 4-point grading scale for deep tendon reflexes.

11. State the vertebral level whose intactness is assessed when eliciting each of these reflexes:

    Biceps reflex _____

    Triceps reflex _____

    Brachioradialis reflex _____

    Quadriceps reflex _____

    Achilles reflex _____

12. List the components of the neurologic recheck examination that are performed routinely on hospital-ized persons being monitored for neurologic deficit.

13. List the 3 areas of assessment on the Glasgow Coma Scale.

14. Describe the gait patterns of the following abnormal gaits:

    Spastic hemiparesis

    Cerebellar ataxia

    Parkinsonian

    Scissors

    Steppage

    Waddling

15. State the type of reflex response you would expect to see with an upper motor neuron lesion versus a lower motor neuron lesion.

16. Describe the method of testing the type of reflexes that are also termed *frontal release signs*.

ASSESSMENT VIDEO CRITICAL THINKING QUESTIONS

Discussion answers to these questions are in the Instructor's Manual for *Physical Examination and Health Assessment*, 4th ed.

1. Which cranial nerve and sensory system assessments would you include in a neurologic screening examination?

2. Describe abnormal assessment findings that occur with lower motor neuron dysfunction of cranial nerve VII.

3. How would you modify your techniques when assessing an older adult's sensory system?

4. Which nursing diagnoses are appropriate for individuals with cranial nerve or sensory deficits?

5. Which motor system and reflex assessments would you include in a neurologic screening examination?

6. What abnormal findings may commonly be detected when assessing a child's gait?

7. What findings would you expect to see when assessing gait and balance in an older adult?

8. What techniques can you use to elicit deep tendon reflexes?

Fill in the labels indicated on the following illustrations.

A. Medial view of right hemisphere   B. Coronal section

CONTENTS OF THE CENTRAL NERVOUS SYSTEM

Fill in the name of each cranial nerve, then write S (sensory), M (Motor), or MX (mixed).

REVIEW QUESTIONS

This test is for you and is intended to check your own mastery of the content. The answers are provided in Appendix A.

1. The medical record indicates that a person has an injury to Broca's area. When meeting this person you expect:

   a) difficulty speaking.
   b) receptive aphasia.
   c) visual disturbances.
   d) emotional lability.

2. The control of body temperature is located in:

   a) Wernicke's area.
   b) the thalamus.
   c) the cerebellum.
   d) the hypothalamus.

3. To test for stereognosis, you would:

   a) have the person close his or her eyes, then raise the person's arm and ask the person to describe its location.
   b) touch the person with a tuning fork.
   c) place a coin in the person's hand and ask him or her to identify it.
   d) touch the person with a cold object.

4. During the examination of an infant, use a cotton-tipped applicator to stimulate the anal sphincter. The absence of a response suggests a lesion of:

   a) L2.
   b) T12.
   c) S2.
   d) C5.

5. During a neurologic examination, the tendon reflex fails to appear. Before striking the tendon again, the examiner might use the technique of:

   a) two-point discrimination.
   b) reinforcement.
   c) vibration.
   d) graphesthesia.

6. Cerebellar function is assessed by which of the following tests?

   a) muscle size and strength
   b) cranial nerve examination
   c) coordination—hop on one foot
   d) spinothalamic test

7. To elicit a Babinski reflex:

   a) gently tap the Achilles tendon.
   b) stroke the lateral aspect of the sole of the foot from heel to the ball.
   c) present a noxious odor to a person.
   d) observe the person walking heel to toe.

8. A positive Babinski sign is:

   a) dorsiflexion of the big toe and fanning of all toes.
   b) plantar flexion of the big toe with a fanning of all toes.
   c) the expected response in healthy adults.
   d) withdrawal of the stimulated extremity from the stimulus.

9. The cremasteric response:

   a) is positive when disease of the pyramidal tract is present.
   b) is positive when the ipsilateral testicle elevates upon stroking of the inner aspect of the thigh.
   c) is a reflex of the receptors in the muscles of the abdomen.
   d) is not a valid neurologic examination.

10. To examine for the function of the trigeminal nerve in an infant, you would:

    a) startle the baby.
    b) hold an object within the child's line of vision.
    c) pinch the nose of the child.
    d) offer the baby a bottle.

11. Senile tremors may resemble parkinsonism, except that senile tremors do not include:

    a) nodding the head as if responding yes or no.
    b) rigidity and weakness of voluntary movement.
    c) tremor of the hands.
    d) tongue protrusion.

12. People who have Parkinson's disease usually have which of the following characteristic styles of speech?

    a) a garbled manner
    b) loud, urgent
    c) slow, monotonous
    d) word confusion

Match column A with column B.

Column A—Cranial nerve

13. _____ Olfactory

14. _____ Optic

15. _____ Oculomotor

16. _____ Trochlear

17. _____ Trigeminal

18. _____ Abducens

19. _____ Facial

20. _____ Acoustic

21. _____ Glossopharyngeal

22. _____ Vagus

23. _____ Spinal

24. _____ Hypoglossal

Column B—Function

a. movement of the tongue

b. vision

c. lateral movement of the eyes

d. hearing and equilibrium

e. talking, swallowing, carotid sinus, and carotid reflex

f. smell

g. extraocular movement, pupil constriction, down and inward movement of the eye

h. mastication and sensation of face, scalp, cornea

i. phonation, swallowing, taste posterior 1/3 of tongue

j. movement of trapezius and sternomastoid muscles

k. down and inward movement of the eye

l. taste anterior 2/3 of tongue, close eyes

SKILLS LABORATORY/CLINICAL SETTING

You are now ready for the clinical component of the neurologic system. The purpose of the clinical component is to practice the regional examination on a peer in the skills laboratory or a patient in the clinical setting and to achieve the following.

CLINICAL OBJECTIVES

1. Demonstrate knowledge of the symptoms related to the neurologic system by obtaining a regional health history from a peer or patient.

2. Demonstrate examination of the neurologic system by assessing the cranial nerves, cerebellar function, sensory system, motor system, and deep tendon reflexes.

3. Record the history and physical examination findings accurately, reach an assessment of the health state, and develop a plan of care.

INSTRUCTIONS

Gather all equipment for a complete neurologic examination. Wash your hands. Practice the steps of the exam on a peer or a patient in the clinical setting, giving appropriate instructions as you proceed. Record your findings using the regional write-up sheet that follows. The first section is intended as a worksheet; the last page is intended for your narrative summary recording using the SOAP format.

NOTES

REGIONAL WRITE-UP—NEUROLOGIC SYSTEM

Date _____

Patient _____ Age _____ Sex _____ Occupation _____

Examiner _____

I. Health History

	No	Yes, explain
1. Any unusual frequent or unusually severe **headaches**?		
2. Ever had any **head injury**?		
3. Ever feel **dizziness**?		
4. Ever had any **convulsions**?		
5. Any **tremors** in hands or face?		
6. Any **weakness** in any body part?		
7. Any problem with **coordination**?		
8. Any **numbness or tingling**?		
9. Any problem **swallowing**?		
10. Any problem **speaking**?		
11. Past history of stroke, spinal cord injury, meningitis, congenital defect, alcoholism?		
12. Any environmental/occupational hazards, e.g., insecticides?		

II. Physical Examination

A. Cranial nerves

I _____

II _____

III, IV, VI _____

V _____

VII _____

VIII _____

IX, X _____

XI _____

XII _____

B. Motor system

1. Muscles

   Size, strength, tone _____

   Involuntary movements _____

2. Cerebellar function

   Gait _____

   Romberg test _____

   Rapid alternative movements _____

   Finger-to-finger test _____

   Finger-to-nose test _____

   Heel-to-shin test _____

C. Sensory system

1. Spinothalamic tract

Pain _____

Temperature _____

Light touch _____

2. Posterior column tract

Vibration _____

Position (kinesthesia) _____

Tactile discrimination _____

    Stereognosis _____

    Graphesthesia _____

    Two-point discrimination _____

D. Reflexes

	Bi	Tri	BR	P	A	PL($\uparrow$/$\downarrow$)	Abd	Cre	Bab
R									
L									

0 = absent; 1+ = hypoactive; 2+ = normal; 3+ = hyperactive;
4+ = hyperactive with clonus; $\uparrow$ dorsiflexion; $\downarrow$ plantar flexion

REGIONAL WRITE-UP—NEUROLOGIC SYSTEM

Summarize your findings using the SOAP format.

Subjective (Reason for seeking care, health history)

Objective (Physical exam findings)

Record reflexes on diagram below.

Assessment (Assessment of health state or problem, diagnosis)

Plan (Diagnostic evaluation, follow-up care, patient teaching)

CHAPTER 24

Male Genitalia

PURPOSE

This chapter helps you to learn the structure and function of the male genitalia; to learn the methods of inspection and palpation of these structures; and to record the assessment accurately.

READING ASSIGNMENT

Jarvis, *Physical Examination and Health Assessment*, 4th ed., Chapter 24, pp. 721-748.

AUDIO-VISUAL ASSIGNMENT

Jarvis, *Saunders Video Series: Physical Examination and Health Assessment: Male Genitalia*

GLOSSARY

Study the following terms after completing the reading assignment. You should be able to cover the definition on the right and define the term out loud.

Chancre .... red, round, superficial ulcer with a yellowish serous discharge that is a sign of syphilis

Condylomata acuminata .... soft, pointed, fleshy papules that occur on the genitalia and are caused by the human papillomavirus (HPV)

Cryptorchidism .... undescended testes

Cystitis .... inflammation of the urinary bladder

Epididymis .... structure composed of coiled ducts located over the superior and posterior surface of the testes, which stores sperm

Epispadias .... congenital defect in which urethra opens on the dorsal (upper) side of penis instead of at the tip

Hernia .... weak spot in abdominal muscle wall (usually in area of inguinal canal or femoral canal) through which a loop of bowel may protrude

Herpes genitalis .... a sexually transmitted disease characterized by clusters of small painful vesicles, caused by a virus

Hydrocele .... cystic fluid in tunica vaginalis surrounding testis

Hypospadias .... congenital defect in which urethra opens on the ventral (under) side of penis rather than at the tip

Orchitis .... acute inflammation of testis, usually associated with mumps

Paraphimosis .... foreskin is retracted and fixed behind the glans penis

Peyronie's disease .... nontender, hard plaques on the surface of penis, associated with painful bending of penis during erection

Phimosis .... foreskin is advanced and tightly fixed over the glans penis

Prepuce .... (foreskin) the hood or flap of skin over the glans penis that often is surgically removed after birth by circumcision

Priapism .... prolonged, painful erection of penis without sexual desire

Spermatic cord .... collection of vas deferens, blood vessels, lymphatics, and nerves that ascends along the testis and through the inguinal canal into the abdomen

Spermatocele .... retention cyst in epididymis filled with milky fluid that contains sperm

Torsion .... sudden twisting of spermatic cord; a surgical emergency

Varicocele .... dilated tortuous varicose veins in the spermatic cord

Vas deferens .... duct carrying sperm from the epididymis through the abdomen and then into the urethra

STUDY GUIDE

After completing the reading assignment and the audio-visual assignment, you should be able to answer the following questions in the space provided.

1. Describe the function of the cremaster muscle.

2. Identify the structures that provide transport of sperm.

3. Describe the significance of the inguinal canal and the femoral canal.

4. List the pros and cons of circumcision of the male newborn.

5. Discuss ways of creating an environment that will provide psychologic comfort for the man and the examiner during examination of male genitalia.

6. List teaching points to include with the teaching of testicular self-examination.

7. Discuss the rationale for making certain that testes have descended in the male infant.

8. Contrast the physical appearance and clinical significance of these scrotal lumps:

   Epididymitis

   Varicocele

   Spermatocele

   Testicular tumor

   Hydrocele

9. Contrast the anatomic course and the clinical significance of these hernias:

   Indirect inguinal

Direct inguinal

Femoral

ASSESSMENT VIDEO CRITICAL THINKING QUESTIONS

Discussion answers to these questions are in the Instructor's Manual for *Physical Examination and Health Assessment*, 4th ed.

1. Which presenting symptoms are associated with abnormalities of the male genitalia?

2. What abnormal findings may be detected during inspection of the penis?

3. How do genitalia assessment findings in a male infant compare to those in a male adolescent?

Fill in the labels indicated on the following illustrations.

STRUCTURES OF THE INGUINAL AREA

REVIEW QUESTIONS

This test is for you and is intended to check your own mastery of the content. Answers are provided in Appendix A.

1. The examiner is going to inspect and palpate for a hernia. During this exam, the man is instructed to:

   a) hold his breath during palpation.
   b) cough after the examiner has gently inserted the exam finger into the rectum.
   c) bear down when the examiner's finger is at the inguinal canal.
   d) relax in a supine position while the exam finger is inserted into the canal.

2. During examination of the scrotum, a normal finding would be:

   a) The left testicle is firmer to palpation than the right.
   b) The left testicle is larger than the right.
   c) The left testicle hangs lower than the right.
   d) The left testicle is more tender to palpation than the right.

3. H. T. has come to the clinic for a follow-up visit. Six months ago, he was started on a new medication. The class of medication is most likely to cause impotence as a side effect; therefore, medication classes explored by the nurse are:

   a) antipyretics.
   b) bronchodilators.
   c) corticosteroids.
   d) antihypertensives.

4. Prostatic hypertrophy occurs frequently in older men. The symptoms that may indicate this problem are:

   a) polyuria and urgency.
   b) dysuria and oliguria.
   c) straining, loss of force, and sense of residual urine.
   d) foul-smelling urine and dysuria.

5. A 64-year-old man has come for a health examination. A normal, age-related change in the scrotum would be:

   a) testicular atrophy.
   b) testicular hypertrophy.
   c) pendulous scrotum.
   d) increase in scrotal rugae.

6. During palpation of the testes, the normal finding would be:

   a) firm to hard, and rough.
   b) nodular.
   c) 2 to 3 cm long by 2 cm wide and firm.
   d) firm, rubbery, and smooth.

7. A 20-year-old man has indicated that he does not perform testicular self-examination. One of the facts that should be shared with him is that testicular cancer, though rare, does occur in men aged:

   a) under 15.
   b) 15 to 34.
   c) 35 to 55.
   d) 55 and older.

8. During the examination of a full-term new-born male, a finding requiring investigation would be:

   a) absent testes.
   b) meatus centered at the tip of the penis.
   c) wrinkled scrotum.
   d) penis 2 to 3 cm in length.

9. During transillumination of a scrotum, you note a nontender mass that transilluminates with a red glow. This finding is suggestive of:

   a) scrotal hernia.
   b) scrotal edema.
   c) orchitis.
   d) hydrocele.

10. How sensitive to pressure are normal testes?

    a) somewhat
    b) not at all
    c) left is more sensitive than right
    d) only when inflammation is present

11. The congenital displacement of the urethral meatus to the inferior surface of the penis is:

    a) hypospadias.
    b) epispadias.
    c) hypoesthesia.
    d) hypophysis.

12. An adhesion of the prepuce to the head of the penis, making it impossible to retract, is:

    a) paraphimosis.
    b) phimosis.
    c) smegma.
    d) dyschezia.

13. The first physical sign associated with puberty in boys is:

    a) height spurt.
    b) penis lengthening.
    c) sperm production.
    d) pubic hair development.
    e) testes enlargement.

14. Write a narrative account of an assessment of male genitalia with normal findings.

SKILLS LABORATORY/CLINICAL SETTING

You are now ready for the clinical component of the male genitalia exam. Because of the need to maintain personal privacy, it is likely you will not practice this examination on a classmate. Your practice likely will be with a teaching mannequin in the skills laboratory or with a male in the clinical setting. Before you proceed, discuss the feelings that may be experienced by the man and the examiner and methods to increase the comfort of both. Make sure you have discussed the steps of the examination with your instructor before examining a patient.

CLINICAL OBJECTIVES

1. Demonstrate knowledge of the signs and symptoms related to the male genitalia by obtaining a pertinent health history.

2. Inspect and palpate the penis and scrotum.

3. Palpate the inguinal region for hernia.

4. Teach testicular self-examination.

5. Record the history and physical examination findings accurately, reach an assessment of the health state, and develop a plan of care.

INSTRUCTIONS

Prepare the examination setting and gather your equipment. Wash your hands; wear gloves during the examination. Practice the steps of the exam on a male in the clinical setting, giving appropriate instructions as you proceed. Record your findings using the regional write-up sheet that follows. The front of the page is intended as a worksheet; the back of the page is intended for your narrative summary recording using the SOAP format.

Note the student performance checklist that follows the regional write-up sheet. It lists the essential behaviors you should display as an examiner, and it may be used by your clinical instructor to evaluate your clinical teaching of testicular self-examination.

Jarvis, Carolyn: PHYSICAL EXAMINATION AND HEALTH ASSESSMENT, Fourth Edition,
Student Laboratory Manual. Copyright © 2004, 2000, 1996, Elsevier Inc. All rights reserved.

NOTES

REGIONAL WRITE-UP—MALE GENITALIA

Date _____

Patient _____ Age _____ Sex _____ Occupation _____

Examiner _____

I. Health History

	No	Yes, explain
1. Any urinary **frequency, urgency,** or wakening during night to urinate?		
2. Any **pain** or **burning** with urinating?		
3. Any **trouble starting urine stream**?		
4. Urine **color cloudy** or **foul-smelling**?		
Red-tinged or **bloody**?		
5. Any **problem controlling your urine**?		
6. Any **pain** or **sores** on penis?		
7. Any **lump** in testicles or scrotum?		
Do you perform testicular self-exam?		
8. In relationship now involving intercourse?		
Use a contraceptive? Which one?		
9. Any contact with partner who has sexually transmitted disease?		

II. Physical Examination

A. Inspect and palpate penis

Skin condition _____

Glans _____

Urethral meatus _____

Shaft _____

B. Inspect and palpate the scrotum

Skin condition _____

Testes _____

Spermatic cord _____

Transillumination (if indicated) _____

C. Inspect and palpate for hernia

Inguinal canal _____

Femoral area _____

D. Palpate inguinal lymph nodes

E. Teach testicular self-examination

REGIONAL WRITE-UP—MALE GENITALIA

Summarize your findings using the SOAP format.

Subjective (Reason for seeking care, health history)

Objective (Physical exam findings)

Assessment (Assessment of problem, diagnosis)

Plan (Diagnostic evaluation, follow-up care, patient teaching)

STUDENT PERFORMANCE CHECKLIST

TEACHING TESTICULAR SELF-EXAMINATION (TSE)

	S	U	Comments

I. Cognitive
    1. Explain:
      a. why testicles are examined			

b. who should perform TSE			
c. frequency of testicular exam			
2. Describe the technique			
II. Performance			
1. Explains to male need for TSE			
2. Instructs male on technique of TSE by:			
a. describing method of palpating testicles			
b. describing normal findings			
c. describing abnormal findings to look for			
3. Instructs male to report unusual findings promptly			

CHAPTER 25

Anus, Rectum, and Prostate

PURPOSE

This chapter helps you to learn the structure and function of the anus and rectum and the male prostate gland; the methods of inspection and palpation of these structures; and how to record the assessment accurately.

READING ASSIGNMENT

Jarvis, *Physical Examination and Health Assessment,* 4th ed., Chapter 25, pp. 749-764.

AUDIO-VISUAL ASSIGNMENT

Jarvis, *Saunders Video Series: Physical Examination and Health Assessment: Male Genitalia*

GLOSSARY

Study the following terms after completing the reading assignment. You should be able to cover the definition on the right and define the term out loud.

Fissure .... painful longitudinal tear in tissue, e.g., in the superficial mucosa at the anal margin

Hemorrhoid .... flabby papules of skin or mucous membrane in the anal region caused by a varicose vein of the hemorrhoidal plexus

Melena .... blood in the stool

Pruritus .... itching or burning sensation in the skin

Steatorrhea .... excessive fat in the stool as in gastrointestinal malabsorption of fat

Valves of Houston .... one of three semilunar transverse folds that cross one-half the circumference of the rectal lumen

STUDY GUIDE

After completing the reading assignment and the audio-visual assignment, you should be able to answer the following questions in the spaces provided.

1. State the length of the anal canal and the rectum in the adult, and describe the location of these structures in the lower abdomen.

2. Describe the size, shape, and location of the male prostate gland.

3. List a few examples of high-fiber foods of the soluble type and of the insoluble type; what advantages do these foods have for the body?

4. List screening measures that are recommended for early detection of colon/rectal cancer; of prostate cancer.

5. State the method of promoting anal sphincter relaxation in order to aid palpation of the anus and rectum.

6. Describe the normal physical characteristics of the prostate gland that would be assessed by palpation:

Size

Shape

Surface

Consistency

Mobility

Sensitivity

7. Describe the physical appearance and clinical significance of pilondial cyst, and anorectal fistula.

8. Define the condition *benign prostatic hypertrophy*, list the usual symptoms the man experiences with this condition, and describe the physical characteristics.

ASSESSMENT VIDEO CRITICAL THINKING QUESTIONS

Discussion answers to these questions are in the Instructor's Manual for *Physical Examination and Health Assessment.*

1. Describe abnormal findings that may be noted on inspection of the perianal canal of an infant or child.

Fill in the labels indicated on the following illustration.

REVIEW QUESTIONS

This test is for you and is intended to check your own mastery of the content. Answers are provided in Appendix A.

1. The gastrocolic reflex is:

   a) a peristaltic wave.
   b) the passage of meconium in the newborn.
   c) another term for borborygmi.
   d) reverse peristalsis.

2. The incidence of benign prostatic hypertrophy (BPH) is highest among:

   a) European Americans.
   b) African Americans.
   c) Hispanics.
   d) Asians.

3. Select the best description of the anal canal.

   a) a 12-cm-long portion of the large intestine
   b) under involuntary control of the parasympathetic nervous system
   c) a 3.8-cm-long outlet of the gastrointestinal tract
   d) an S-shaped portion of the colon

4. While good nutrition is important for everyone, foods believed to help reduce risk of colon cancer are:

   a) high in fiber.
   b) low in fat.
   c) high in protein.
   d) high in carbohydrate.

5. Which finding in the prostate gland suggests prostate cancer?

   a) symmetrical smooth enlargement
   b) extreme tenderness to palpation
   c) boggy soft enlargement
   d) diffuse hardness

6. The bulbourethral gland is assessed:

   a) during an examination of a female patient.
   b) during an examination of both male and female patients.
   c) during an examination of a male patient.
   d) cannot be assessed with a rectal examination.

7. Inspection of stool is an important part of the rectal examination. Normal stool is:

   a) black in color and tarry in consistency.
   b) brown in color and soft in consistency.
   c) clay colored and dry in consistency.
   d) varies depending upon the individual's diet.

8. Which symptoms suggest benign prostatic hypertrophy?

   a) weight loss and bone pain
   b) fever, chills, urinary frequency, and urgency
   c) difficulty initiating urination and weak stream
   d) dark, tarry stools

9. A false positive may occur on fecal occult blood tests of the stool if the person has ingested significant amounts of:

   a) red meat
   b) candies with red dye #2
   c) cranberry juice
   d) red beets

10. Write a narrative account of a rectal assessment with normal findings.

SKILLS LABORATORY/CLINICAL SETTING

You are now ready for the clinical component of the rectal examination. This regional examination usually is combined with the examination of the male genitalia or with examination of the female genitalia.

CLINICAL OBJECTIVES

1. Demonstrate knowledge of the signs and symptoms related to the rectal area by obtaining a pertinent health history.

2. Inspect and palpate the perianal region.

3. Test any stool specimen for occult blood.

4. Record the history and physical examination findings accurately.

INSTRUCTIONS

Prepare the examination setting and gather your equipment. Wash your hands; wear gloves during the examination; wash hands again after removing gloves. Practice the steps of the exam on a patient in the clinical setting, giving appropriate instructions as you proceed. Record your findings using the regional write-up sheet that follows. Note that only the worksheet is included in this chapter. Your narrative summary recording using the SOAP format can be included with the narrative summary of the genitalia.

NOTES

REGIONAL WRITE-UP—ANUS, RECTUM, AND PREOSTATE GLAND   Date _____

Patient _____ Age _____ Sex _____ Occupation _____

Examiner _____

I. Health History

	No	Yes, explain
1. Bowels move **regularly**? How often?		
Usual color? Hard or soft?		
2. Any **change** in usual bowel habits?		
3. Ever had **black or bloody stool**?		
4. Take any medications?		
5. Any **rectal itching, pain, or hemorrhoids**?		
6. Any family history of **colon/rectal polyps or cancer**?		
7. Describe usual amount of high-fiber foods in diet.		

II. Physical Examination

A. Inspect the perianal area
Skin condition _____
Sacrococcygeal area _____
Note skin integrity while patient performs Valsalva maneuver _____

B. Palpate anus and rectum
Anal sphincter _____
Anal canal _____
Rectal wall _____
Prostate gland (for males)
  Size _____
  Shape _____
  Surface _____
  Consistency _____
  Mobility _____
  Any tenderness _____
Cervix (for females) _____

C. Examination of stool
Visual inspection _____
Test for occult blood _____

CHAPTER 26

Female Genitalia

This chapter helps you to learn the structure and function of the female genitalia; the methods of inspection and palpation of the internal and external structures; the procedures for collection of cytological specimens; and to record the assessment accurately.

READING ASSIGNMENT

Jarvis, *Physical Examination and Health Assessment*, 4th ed., Chapter 26, pp. 765-802.

AUDIO-VISUAL ASSIGNMENT

Jarvis, *Saunders Video Series: Physical Examination and Health Assessment: Female Genitalia*

GLOSSARY

Study the following terms after completing the reading assignment. You should be able to cover the definition on the right and define the term out loud.

Adnexa .... accessory organs of the uterus, i.e., ovaries and fallopian tubes

Amenorrhea .... absence of menstruation; termed secondary amenorrhea when menstruation has begun and then ceases; most common cause is pregnancy

Bartholin's glands .... vestibular glands, located on either side of the vaginal orifice, that secrete a clear lubricating mucus during intercourse

Bloody show .... dislodging of thick cervical mucus plug at end of pregnancy, which is a sign of beginning of labor

Caruncle .... small, deep red mass protruding from urethral meatus, usually due to urethritis

Chadwick's sign .... bluish discoloration of cervix that occurs normally in pregnancy at 6 to 8 weeks' gestation

Chancre .... red, round, superficial ulcer with a yellowish serous discharge that is a sign of syphilis

Clitoris .... small, elongated erectile tissue in the female, located at anterior juncture of labia minora

Cystocele .... prolapse of urinary bladder and its vaginal mucosa into the vagina with straining or standing

Dysmenorrhea .... abdominal cramping and pain associated with menstruation

Dyspareunia .... painful intercourse

Dysuria .... painful urination

Endometriosis .... aberrant growths of endometrial tissue scattered throughout pelvis

Fibroid .... (myoma) hard painless nodules in uterine wall that cause uterine enlargement

Gonorrhea .... sexually transmitted disease characterized by purulent vaginal discharge, or may have no symptoms

Hegar's sign .... softening of cervix that is a sign of pregnancy, occuring at 10 to 12 weeks' gestation

Hematuria .... red-tinged or bloody urination

Hymen .... membranous fold of tissue partly closing vaginal orifice

Leukorrhea .... whitish or yellowish discharge from vaginal orifice

Menarche .... onset of first menstruation, usually between 11 and 13 years of age

Menopause .... cessation of the menses, usually occurring around 48 to 51 years

Menorrhagia .... excessively heavy menstrual flow

Multipara .... condition of having two or more pregnancies

Nullipara .... condition of first pregnancy

Papanicolaou test .... painless test used to detect cervical cancer

Polyp .... cervical polyp is bright red, soft, pedunculated growth emerging from os

Rectouterine pouch .... (cul-de-sac of Douglas) deep recess formed by the peritoneum between the rectum and cervix

Rectocele .... prolapse of rectum and its vaginal mucosa into vagina with straining or standing

Salpingitis .... inflammation of fallopian tubes

Skene's glands .... paraurethral glands

Vaginitis .... inflammation of vagina

Vulva .... external genitalia of female

STUDY GUIDE

After completing the reading assignment and the audio-visual assignment, you should be able to answer the following questions in the spaces provided.

1. List the external structures of the female genitalia.

2. Describe the size, shape, and location of the internal structures of the female genitalia.

3. Outline the changes observed during the perimenopausal period.

4. Discuss ways of creating an environment that will provide psychologic comfort for both the woman and practitioner during the female genitalia examination.

5. Discuss selection, preparation, and insertion of the vaginal speculum.

6. Describe the appearance or *sketch* these normal variations of the cervix and os:

Nulliparous _____

Parous _____

Stellate lacerations _____

Cervical eversion _____

Nabothian cysts _____

7. List the steps in procedure of obtaining these specimens:

Vaginal pool

Cervical scrape using spatula

Endocervical specimen using cytobrush

8. When applying acetic acid (white vinegar) to the cervix and vaginal mucosa, list the normal response and the response suggesting infection.

9. Discuss the procedure and rationale for bimanual examination and list normal findings for cervix, uterus, adnexa.

10. Discuss infection control precautions during examination of female genitalia and procuring of specimens.

11. Describe the appearance or *sketch* the appearance of the following abnormalities of the cervix:

Chadwick's sign

Erosion

Polyp

Carcinoma

12. List the characteristics of vaginal discharge associated with the following conditions of vaginitis:

Candidiasis

Trichomoniasis

Bacterial vaginosis

Chlamydia

Gonorrhea

14. Differentiate the signs and symptoms of these conditions of adnexal enlargement:

Ectopic pregnancy

Ovarian cyst

ASSESSMENT VIDEO CRITICAL THINKING QUESTIONS

Discussion answers to these questions are in the Instructor's Manual for *Physical Examination and Health Assessment*, 4th ed.

1. What presenting complaint would lead you to assess the female genitalia?

2. How may you adapt the female genitalia assessment to allow for health education?

3. How do normal genitalia examination findings differ between nulliparous women and parous women who gave birth vaginally?

4. What normal and abnormal findings may commonly be detected by a rectovaginal examination?

Fill in the labels indicated on the following illustrations.

ANTERIOR VIEW OF ADNEXA

REVIEW QUESTIONS

This test is for you and is intended to check your own mastery of the content. Answers are provided in Appendix A.

1. Vaginal lubrication is provided during intercourse by:

    a) the labia minora.
    b) sebaceous follicles.
    c) Skene's glands.
    d) Bartholin's glands.

2. A young woman has come for her first gynecologic examination. Since she has not had any children, the examiner would expect the cervical os to appear:

    a) smooth and circular.
    b) irregular and slit like.
    c) irregular and circular.
    d) smooth and enlarged.

3. A woman has come for an examination because of a missed menstrual period and a positive home pregnancy test. Examination reveals a cervix that appears cyanotic. This is referred to as:

    a) Goodell's sign.
    b) Hegar's sign.
    c) Tanner's sign.
    d) Chadwick's sign.

4. During the examination of the genitalia of a 70-year-old woman a normal finding would be:

    a) hypertrophy of the mons pubis.
    b) increase in vaginal secretions.
    c) thin and sparse pubic hair.
    d) bladder prolapse.

5. For a woman, history of her mother's health during pregnancy is important. A medication that requires frequent follow-up is:

    a) corticosteroid.
    b) theophylline.
    c) diethylstilbestrol.
    d) aminoglycoside.

6. A woman has come for health care complaining of a thick, white discharge with intense itching. These symptoms are suggestive of:

    a) atrophic vaginitis.
    b) trichomoniasis.
    c) chlamydia.
    d) candidiasis.

7. To prepare the vaginal speculum for insertion, the examiner:

    a) lubricates it with a water-soluble lubricant.
    b) lubricates it with petrolatum.
    c) warms it under the light, then inserts it into the vagina.
    d) lubricates it with warm water.

8. To insert the speculum as comfortably as possible, the examiner:

    a) opens the speculum slightly and inserts in an upward direction.
    b) presses the introitus down with one hand and inserts the blades obliquely with the other.
    c) spreads the labia with one hand, inserts the closed speculum horizontally with the other.
    d) pushes down on the introitus and inserts the speculum in an upward direction.

9. Before withdrawing the speculum, the examiner swabs the cervix with a swab soaked in acetic acid. This exam is done to assess for:

   a) herpes simplex virus.
   b) contact dermatitis.
   c) human papilloma virus.
   d) carcinoma.

10. Select the best description of the uterus.

    a) anteverted, round asymmetrical organ
    b) pear-shaped, thick-walled organ flattened anteroposteriorly
    c) retroverted, almond-shaped asymmetrical organ
    d) midposition, thick-walled oval organ

11. In placing a finger on either side of the cervix and moving it side to side, you are assessing:

    a) the diameter of the fallopian tube.
    b) cervical motion tenderness.
    c) the ovaries.
    d) the uterus.

12. Which of the following is (are) normal, common finding(s) on inspection and palpation of the vulva and perineum?

    a) labia majora that are wide apart and gaping
    b) palpable Bartholin's glands
    c) clear, thin discharge from paraurethral glands
    d) bulging at introitus during Valsalva maneuver

13. Which of the following is the most common bacterial sexually transmitted disease in the United States?

    a) chlamydia
    b) gonorrhea
    c) trichomoniasis
    d) syphilis
    e) bacterial vaginosis

14. Write a narrative account of an assessment of female genitalia with normal findings.

SKILLS LABORATORY/CLINICAL SETTING

You are now ready for the clinical component of the female genitalia exam. Because of the need to maintain personal privacy, it is likely you will not practice this examination on a peer. Your practice likely will be with a teaching mannequin in the skills laboratory or with a woman in the clinical setting under the guidance of a preceptor. Before you proceed, discuss the feelings that may be experienced by the woman and examiner and methods to increase the comfort of both. With your instructor, discuss methods of positioning the woman, steps in using the vaginal speculum, steps in procuring specimens, and methods of infection control precautions.

CLINICAL OBJECTIVES

1. Demonstrate knowledge of the signs and symptoms related to the female genitalia by obtaining a pertinent health history.

2. Demonstrate measures to increase the woman's comfort before and during the examination.

3. Demonstrate knowledge of infection control precautions before, during, and after the examination.

4. Inspect and palpate the external genitalia.

5. Using the vaginal speculum, gather materials for cytologic study.

6. Inspect and palpate the internal genitalia.

7. Record the history and physical examination findings accurately, reach an assessment of the health state, and develop a plan of care.

INSTRUCTIONS

Prepare the examination setting and gather your equipment. Collect the health history before the woman disrobes for the examination. Wash your hands; wear gloves during the examination; wash hands again after removing gloves. Practice the steps of the exam on a woman in the clinical setting, giving appropriate instructions as you proceed. Record your findings using the regional write-up sheet that follows. The first section is intended as a worksheet; the last page is intended for your narrative summary recording using the SOAP format. Collection of data for the rectal examination is usually combined with the examination of female genitalia; see Chapter 25 for the regional write-up sheet for the rectal exam.

NOTES

REGIONAL WRITE-UP—FEMALE GENITALIA

Date _____

Patient _____ Age _____ Sex _____ Occupation _____

Examiner _____

I. Health History

	No	Yes, explain

1. Date of **last menstrual period**? _____ _____

   Age at first period? Usual cycle? _____ _____

   Duration? Usual amount of flow? _____ _____

   Any pain or cramps with period? _____ _____

2. Ever been **pregnant**? # times? _____ _____

   Describe pregnancy (ies) _____ _____

   Any complications? _____ _____

3. Periods slowed down or **stopped**? _____ _____

4. How often has **gynecologic checkup**? _____ _____

   Date of last Pap test? Results? _____ _____

5. Any problems with **urinating**? _____ _____

6. Any unusual **vaginal discharge**? _____ _____

7. **Sores** or **lesions** in genitals? _____ _____

8. In relationship now involving intercourse? _____ _____

9. Use a contraceptive? Which one? _____ _____

10. Any contact with partner who has sexually transmitted disease? _____ _____

11. Any precautions to reduce risk of STDs? _____ _____

12. Taking any medications? _____ _____

    Any hormone therapy? _____ _____

II. Physical Examination
A. Inspect external genitalia
Skin color and characteristics _____

Hair distribution _____

Symmetry _____

Clitoris _____

Labia _____

Urethral opening _____

Vaginal opening _____

Perineum _____

B. Palpate external genitalia
Skene's glands _____
Bartholin's glands _____
Perineum _____
Assess perineal muscle strength _____
Assess for vaginal wall bulging or urinary incontinence _____
Discharge and characteristics _____

C. Speculum examination
Inspect cervix and os
    Color _____
    Position _____
    Size _____
    Surface _____
    Discharge and characteristics _____
Obtain cervical smears and cultures _____
    Vaginal pool
    Cervical scrape
    Endocervical specimen
    Other (if indicated)
Complete acetic acid wash
Inspect vaginal wall as speculum is removed _____

D. Bimanual examination
Cervix
    Consistency _____
    Mobility _____
    Tenderness with motion _____
Uterus
    Size and shape _____
    Consistency _____
    Position _____
    Mobility _____
    Tenderness _____
Adnexa _____
    Able to palpate? (Be honest.) _____
    Size and shape of ovaries _____
    Tenderness _____
    Masses _____
Rectovaginal examination

REGIONAL WRITE-UP—FEMALE GENITALIA

Summarize your findings using the SOAP format.

Subjective (Reason for seeking care, health history)

Objective (Physical exam findings)   Record findings on diagram below.

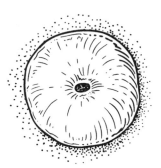

Assessment (Assessment of health state or problem, diagnosis)

Plan (Diagnostic evaluation, follow-up care, patient teaching)

CHAPTER 27

The Pregnant Female

READING ASSIGNMENT

Jarvis, *Physical Examination and Health Assessment,* 4th ed., Chapter 27, pp. 803-834.

AUDIO-VISUAL ASSIGNMENT

GLOSSARY

Study the following terms after completing the reading assignment. You should be able to cover the definition on the right and define the term out loud.

Amniocentesis.............................. the transabdominal perforation of the amniotic sac for the purpose of obtaining a sample of amniotic fluid

Antepartum................................. the period occurring before childbirth

Blastocyst .... the fertilized ovum; a specialized layer of cells around the blastocyst becomes the placenta

Chadwick's sign .... bluish/purple discoloration of the cervix during pregnancy due to venous congestion

Chloasma.................................... the "mask of pregnancy"; butterfly-shaped pigmentation of the face

Chorionic villi sampling............ transabdominal or transvaginal sampling of trophoblastic tissue surrounding the gestational sac

Colostrum .... the precursor to milk that contains minerals, proteins, and antibodies

Corpus luteum .... "yellow body" a structure on the surface of the ovary that is formed by the remaining cells in the follicle; it acts as a short-lived endocrine organ that produces progesterone to help maintain the pregnancy in its early stages

Diastasis recti .... separation of the abdominal muscles during pregnancy, returning to normal after pregnancy

Engagement .... when the widest diameter of the presenting part has descended into the pelvic inlet

Fetal lie .... orientation of the fetal spine to the maternal spine

Goodell's sign .... the softening of the cervix due to increased vascularity, congestion, and edema

Hegar's sign .... where the uterus becomes globular in shape, softens, and flexes easily over the cervix

Hyperemesis gravidarum .... severe and debilitating nausea and vomiting that may persist beyond the 14th week of pregnancy and cause dehydration, weight loss, and electrolyte imbalance

Intrapartum .... occurring during labor and delivery

Leopold's maneuver .... external palpation of the maternal abdomen to determine fetal lie, presentation, attitude, and position

Linea nigra .... a median line of the abdomen that becomes pigmented (darkens) during pregnancy

"Morning sickness" .... nausea and vomiting of pregnancy that usually begins between weeks 4 and 6, peaks between weeks 8 and 12, and resolves between weeks 14 and 16

Mucus plug .... mucus that forms a thick barrier in the cervix that is expelled at various times before or during labor

Mutigravida .... a pregnant woman who has previously carried a fetus to the point of viability

Multipara .... a woman who has had two or more viable pregnancies and deliveries

Nägele's rule .... a rule for calculating the estimated date of confinement; subtract 3 months from the first day of the last menstrual period and add 7 days

Pelvimetry .... assessment of the maternal pelvis bones for shape and size

Pica .... a craving for unnatural articles of food, such as cornstarch and ice chips

Position .... the location of a fetal part to the right or left of the maternal pelvis

Postpartum .... the period occurring after delivery

Presentation .... the part of the fetus that is entering the pelvis first

Primagravida .... a woman pregnant for the first time

Primapara .... a woman who has had one pregnancy and delivery

Striae gravidarum .... "stretch marks" that may be seen on the abdomen and breasts (in areas of weight gain) during pregnancy

"VBAC" .... vaginal birth after cesarean section

STUDY GUIDE

After completing the reading assignment and the audio-visual assignment, you should be able to answer the following questions in the spaces provided.

1. Describe the function of the placenta.

2. Using Nägele's rule, calculate the estimated date of confinement if the LMP is August 22.

3. Give examples of the following signs of pregnancy.

   Presumptive:

   Probable:

   Positive:

4. When can serum hCG be detected in maternal blood?

5. Describe three physical and physiological changes that are seen in the:

   First trimester:

   Second trimester:

   Third trimester:

6. Describe the "expected" weight gain during pregnancy.

7. List the major concerns for teenage maternal morbidity and mortality.

8. List at least three risk factors concerning pregnant woman of advanced maternal age.

9. Discuss the importance of how transcultural differences play a role in a woman's pregnancy.

10. List at least three ways in which you as a healthcare provider can be culturally sensitive to a woman during her antepartum, intrapartum, and postpartum periods.

11. True or False: Please circle the best answer.

True	False	A woman who has had a classical uterine incision is a good candidate for a VBAC.
True	False	In early fetal development, the corpus luteum plays no significance.
True	False	A woman who is pregnant for the first time is called a primapara.
True	False	The fetal period begins after the 9th gestational week.
True	False	Preeclampsia is only seen in the third trimester of pregnancy.
True	False	Vaginal bleeding in pregnancy always indicates a miscarriage.
True	False	Cervical incompetence is always accompanied by painful contractions.

12. What is the importance of fetal movement counting, and when should it be initiated?

13. Describe why it is important to ask a pregnant woman if she feels safe in her relationships and environment.

14. Where on this diagram should the fundal height be at the 20th week of gestation? (Please draw on this diagram.)

15. Label the following types of pelvis.

_____

_____

_____

_____

16. Please label, list the order, and describe the purpose of the following _____ maneuvers. (Fill in above blank.)

_____

_____

_____

_____

17. Describe the following for this figure.

Fetal lie: _____

Fetal presentation: _____

Fetal position: _____

18. List the symptoms of preeclampsia.

19. List at least two reasons why fundal height may be small for gestational age.

20. List at least two reasons why fundal height may be large for gestational age.

REVIEW QUESTIONS

This test is for you and is intended to check your own mastery of the content. Answers are provided in Appendix A.

1. Ovulation begins on the:

   a) first day of the menstrual cycle.
   b) 28th day of the menstrual cycle.
   c) 14th day/approximately of the menstrual cycle.

2. Using Nägele's rule, the estimated date of confinement (EDC) if a woman's last menstrual period started on January 13 is:

   a) $1/13 + 7 = 20$ 20-3 months   EDC = October ≈ 29
   b) $1/13 + 10 = 23$ 23-3 months   EDC = October ≈ 18
   c) $1/13 + 14 = 27$ 27-3 months   EDC = September 31

3. A woman comes to the clinic complaining of nausea, fatigue, breast tenderness, urinary frequency, and amenorrhea. These are:

   a) Probable signs of pregnancy.
   b) Positive signs of pregnancy.
   c) Presumptive signs of pregnancy.
   d) Signs of stress.

4. After implantation, what structure makes progesterone to support the pregnancy up until week 10?

   a) corpus luteum
   b) blastocyst
   c) placenta
   d) ovary

5. Approximately 2-3 weeks before labor the woman will experience:

   a) extreme fatigue.
   b) Braxton–Hicks contractions.
   c) lightening.
   d) back pain.

6. Cardiac output in a pregnant woman:

   a) drops dramatically.
   b) remains the same.
   c) increases along with stroke volume.
   d) decreases along with stroke volume.
   e) none of the above.

7. The pregnant adolescent is medically at risk for:

   a) poor weight gain, preeclampsia, thyroiditis, miscarriage.
   b) poor weight gain, preeclampsia, and sexually transmitted diseases.
   c) stress, abuse, inadequate housing, inadequate education.
   d) miscarriage, hypothyroidism, poor weight gain.

8. Women over the age of 35 who desire a pregnancy are at increased risk for:

   a) congenital anomalies.
   b) infertility.
   c) diabetes.
   d) hypertension.
   e) all of the above.

9. Sexually transmitted diseases place the pregnant woman at risk for:

   a) infertility.
   b) premature rupture of membranes.
   c) preterm labor.
   d) preterm delivery.
   e) all of the above.
   f) b, c, and d only.

10. Abdominal pain in the first trimester may be indicative of:

    a) preterm labor.
    b) ectopic pregnancy.
    c) appendicitis.
    d) urinary tract infection.
    e) all of the above.
    f) b, c, and d.

11. A woman at approximately 20 weeks' gestation who is complaining of lower right and/or left quadrant pain may be experiencing:

    a) appendicitis.
    b) constipation.
    c) urinary tract infection.
    d) stretching of the round ligament.
    e) none of the above.

12. You are palpating the maternal abdomen at approximately 35 weeks. Your left hand is on the maternal right, and your right hand is on the maternal left. What maneuver is this?

    a) Leopold's first maneuver
    b) Leopold's second maneuver
    c) Schmidt's third maneuver
    d) Schmidt's second maneuver

13. Fetal heart tones are best auscultated over the fetal:

    a) back.
    b) abdomen.
    c) shoulder.

14. Chadwick's sign is:

    a) softening of the cervix.
    b) rotation of the cervix to the left.
    c) fundus of the uterus tips forward.
    d) a bluish color of the cervix and vaginal walls during early pregnancy.

15. An obstetric ultrasound is done to determine:

   a) thickness of the uterine wall.
   b) fetal position.
   c) placental location.
   d) amniotic fluid volume.
   e) none of the above.
   f) b, c, and d.

16. Write a narrative account of some abnormal findings in pregnancy. List possible causes and consequences to the mother and fetus.

SKILLS LABORATORY/CLINICAL SETTING

You are now ready for the clinical component of the pregnant female exam. Because of the need to maintain personal privacy, it is unlikely you will practice this examination on a peer. Some clinical settings may arrange for pregnant women to participate, or your practice setting may have available a pregnant teaching mannequin that you may use to practice your skills. If you have a pregnant woman available, discuss with her, in the presence of your instructor, the methods of examination that will be used. Maintain her comfort and adequate positioning to prevent maternal dizziness, nausea, and hypotension, and to maintain adequate uterine blood flow.

CLINICAL OBJECTIVES

1. Demonstrate the knowledge of the physical changes related to pregnancy in the first, second, and third trimester.

2. Demonstrate the knowledge and importance of obtaining a pertinent health history during the first prenatal visit.

3. Demonstrate cultural sensitivity during the examination.

4. Inspect and palpate the maternal abdomen for uterine size and fetal position.

5. Demonstrate obtaining fetal heart tones.

6. Record the history and physical examination findings accurately, reach an assessment of the health state, estimated gestational age, fetal position (when appropriate), and develop a plan of care.

INSTRUCTIONS

Prepare the examination setting and gather your equipment. Collect the health history before the woman disrobes for the examination. Calculate the EDC. Wash your hands. Practice the steps of the exam on a woman in the clinical setting, giving appropriate instructions and explanations as you proceed. Record your findings using the regional write-up sheet that follows. The first section is intended as a worksheet; the last page is intended for your narrative summary recording using the SOAP format. See Chapter 26 for the female genital exam.

REGIONAL WRITE-UP – PREGNANT FEMALE

Patient Name _____   Date

PRENATAL HISTORY QUESTIONNAIRE

Having a healthy baby is a special event. Once a baby is born, families take certain precautions to ensure the baby's health and safety. The unborn child deserves similar care.

QUESTIONNAIRE

The following questions will help in the care of your pregnancy. Please answer these questions as well as you can. All answers will remain private. If you need help answering the questions, please ask your health care provider. The first question relates to your family history. The next 7 questions will be about you, your baby's father and both your families. When thinking about your families, please include your child (or unborn baby), mother, father, sisters, brothers, grandparents, aunts, uncles, nieces, nephews, or cousins.

Yes   No   1.   Will you be 35 years or older when the baby is due? Age when due: _____ .

Yes   No   2.   Are you and the baby's father related to each other (e.g., cousins)?

Yes   No   3.   Have you had three or more pregnancies that ended in miscarriage?

Yes   No   4.   Have you or the baby's father had a stillborn baby or a baby who died around the time of delivery?

Yes   No   5.   Do either you or the baby's father have a birth defect or genetic condition such as a baby born with an open spine (spina bifida), a heart defect, or Down's syndrome?

Yes   No   6.   Does anyone in your family or anyone in the baby's father's family have a birth defect or condition that has been diagnosed as genetic or inherited, such as open spine (spina bifida), a heart defect, or Down's Syndrome?

Yes   No   7.   Where your ancestors came from may sometimes give us important information about the health of your baby. Are you or the baby's father from any of the following ethnic/racial groups: Jewish, Black, Asian, Mediterranean (Greek, Italian)?

Yes   No   8.   Have you or the baby's father ever been screened to see if you are carriers of the gene for any of the following: Tay-Sachs, Sickle Cell, Thalassemia?

Sometimes, the unborn baby can be exposed to outside factors that can cause birth defects. The next 8 questions will give us important information about possible exposure to the baby.

Yes   No   9.   Have you had any x-rays during this pregnancy?

Yes   No   10.   Have you had any alcohol during this pregnancy?

11.   Prior to your pregnancy, how often did you drink alcoholic beverages?
☐ Every day   ☐ Less than once a month
☐ At least once a week, not daily   ☐ I do not drink alcoholic beverages.
☐ At least once a month, not weekly

12.   Prior to your pregnancy, about how many alcoholic beverages did you usually have per occasion? (1 = one can of beer, one wine cooler, one glass of wine, or one shot of liquor.)
☐ 3 or more
☐ 1 to 2
☐ I do not drink alcoholic beverages.

Yes   No   13.   Have you taken any over-the-counter, prescription, or "street" drugs during this pregnancy? If yes, list drugs.

_____

_____

Yes   No   14.   Have you ever sought and/or received treatment for alcohol or drug problems? If yes, how long ago?_____

Yes   No   15.   Do you think you are at increased risk of having a baby with a birth defect or genetic disorder?

Yes   No   16.   At any time during the first 2 months of your pregnancy, have you had a rash or a fever of 103° F or greater?

A test for HIV is strongly recommended for all pregnant women, regardless of your responses to the next questions. The test is voluntary. There are two reasons to be tested: [1] New medications are available to reduce the chance of an infected mother passing HIV to her baby; and [2] Most women do not know if they are infected with HIV until late in the disease. Sometimes, other infections can put you and your baby at risk. The following questions will help your health care provider determine other areas for counseling and evaluation.

Yes   No   Unsure   17.   Have you or your sexual partners ever had a sexually transmitted disease (STD or VD) such as chlamydia, gonorrhea, syphilis, or herpes?

Yes   No   Unsure   18.   Have you ever had a serious pelvic infection or pelvic inflammatory disease (PID)?

Yes   No   Unsure   19.   Do you think any of your male sexual partners have ever had sex with other men?

Yes   No   Unsure   20.   Have you or your sexual partners ever used IV street drugs?

Yes   No   Unsure   21.   Have you had sex with two or more partners in the last 12 months?

Yes   No   Unsure   22.   Do you think any of your sexual partners may have HIV or AIDS?

Yes   No   Unsure   23.   Have you or your sexual partners ever had a blood transfusion?

How safe you feel in your daily living gives us important information about risks to you and your baby. Please answer these questions as well as you can. All answers will remain private.

             24.   Do you feel safe....
Yes   No   -   in your personal relationship?
Yes   No   -   within your home?
Yes   No   -   in your own neighborhood?
Yes   No   -   other (specify)_____

Yes   No   25.   Have you ever had your feelings repeatedly hurt, been repeatedly put down, or experienced other kinds of hurting?

Yes   No   26.   Are you being or have you ever been hit, slapped, kicked pushed, or otherwise physically hurt? If yes, by whom?
☐ Husband   ☐ Family member
☐ Ex-husband   ☐ Stranger
☐ Partner   ☐ Other (specify)_____

Yes   No   27.   Are you experiencing or have you ever experienced uncomfortable touching or forced sexual contact? If yes, by whom?
☐ Husband   ☐ Family member
☐ Ex-husband   ☐ Stranger
☐ Partner   ☐ Other (specify)_____

RM/603 REV 6/97

PRENATAL RECORD

DATE	AGE	RACE	RELIGION	OCCUPATION	YRS. ED.	MARITAL STATUS	FATHER OF BABY	FATHER'S WORK PHONE

PHONE-HOME	PHONE-WORK	ADDRESS		REFERRAL-SOURCE	MOTHER'S PRIMARY CARE PROVIDER

GYNECOLOGICAL HISTORY / MEDICAL HISTORY - CONTINUED

GYNECOLOGICAL HISTORY		MEDICAL HISTORY - CONTINUED	
MENARCHE YRS	INTERVAL □ REGULAR □ IRREGULAR DURATION DAYS	CARDIOVASCULAR	
		RESPIRATORY/TB	
✔ IF NEGATIVE-DESCRIBE POSITIVE HISTORY		GI	
PAP HISTORY		GU	
INFERTILITY		METABOLIC	
GYN DISORDER		NEURO	
GYN SURGERY		PSYCH-EMOTIONAL	
DES EXPOSURE		HEPATITIS	
PRIOR CONTRACEPTION		MUSCULOSKELETAL	
BCP W/IN 90 DAYS CONCEP		SKIN DISORDERS	
BREASTS		OTHER DISEASE/DX	
OTHER GYN HX		OPERATIONS	
GONORRHEA		TRANSFUSIONS	
SYPHILIS		ALLERGIES	
CHLAMYDIA		**FAMILY HISTORY - NOTE IF FATHER OF BABY**	
HERPES-SELF/PARTNER		DIABETES	
OTHER STD/HIV		HYPERTENSION	
MEDICAL HISTORY		TWINS	
✔ IF NEGATIVE-DESCRIBE POSITIVE HISTORY		CONGENITAL ANOM	
HEENT		OTHER FAMILY HX	

PREVIOUS PREGNANCIES

NO.	DATE	LENGTH (WKS)	LABOR (HRS)	TYPE DELIVERY	ANES.	SEX	WEIGHT	WHERE DELIVERED	COMPLICATIONS-AP, IP, PP, NEONATAL	OUTCOME/ NAME

PRESENT PREGNANCY HISTORY / PHYSICAL EXAMINATION

PRESENT PREGNANCY HISTORY		PHYSICAL EXAMINATION	DATE
LMP □ NORM □ ABNORM	LNMP EDC + PG TEST TYPE DATE	✔ IF NEGATIVE-DESCRIBE POSITIVE FINDINGS	
PLANNED PREGNANCY/OK?	FATHER SUPPORTIVE?	HEIGHT	
		WEIGHT	
✔ IF NEGATIVE-DESCRIBE POSITIVE HISTORY		B.P.	
NAUSEA/VOMITING		HEENT	
BLEEDING		NECK	
URINARY SX		LUNGS	
VAGINAL DISCHARGE		BREASTS	
INFECTION		HEART	
FEVER/RASH		ABDOMEN	
TOBACCO/SMOKING		NEURO	
ETOH		EXTREMITIES/SKIN	
PHYSICAL/SEXUAL ABUSE		**PELVIC EXAMINATION**	**DATE**
		EXT. GENITALIA	
PATIENT NO.		VAGINA/CERVIX	
		UTERUS-SIZE	
		PELVIS	
PATIENT NAME		ADNEXA	
		BONY PELVIS/ADEQUATE?	
		HEMORRHOIDS	
D.O.B.		PROVIDER SIGNATURE	

FIRST TRIMESTER				DATE	PROBLEMS AND RISK FACTORS
	DATE	WEEKS	EDC/RANGE		
LMP					
LNMP					
OVU/CONCEP					
FIRST EXAM					
+ HCG URINE					
+ HCG SERUM					
FHT DOPPLER					
FHT FETOSCOPE					
FM					
ULTRASOUND					
ULTRASOUND					
ULTRASOUND					

ANTICIPATORY GUIDANCE

FIRST TRIMESTER	SECOND TRIMESTER	THIRD TRIMESTER

CLINIC PROCEDURES/OUTLINE PRENATAL CARE
HIV COUNSELING/TESTING
NUTRITION
VITAMINS/MINERALS
DENTAL/VISION CARE
WEIGHT GAIN
SEAT BELTS
EXERCISE
PRENATAL DIAGNOSIS
HAZARDS: SMOKING, ETOH, DRUGS, OVERHEATING, CATS,
      RAW MEAT, UNPASTEURIZED MILK
DISCOMFORTS/RELIEF MEASURES
WARNING SIGNS: BLEEDING, CRAMPS, ABDOMINAL
             PAINS, DYSURIA, ETC.
BROCHURES
	FETAL DEVELOPMENT/QUICKENING
	FAMILY/FATHER/SIBLINGS
	HOSPITAL PRE-ADMISSION/TOUR?
	FEEDING PLANS (BREAST/BOTTLE)
	EXERCISES/BODY MECHANICS
	WARNING SIGNS: SROM, BLEEDING, PRE-TERM LABOR
	BABY'S CARE PROVIDER _____
	      NEWBORN CARE/ROOMING-IN
	      CIRCUMCISION
	BROCHURES
	PRENATAL CLASSES
	SUPPORT PERSON _____
	BIRTH PLANS/OPTIONS
	SEXUALITY
		DISCOMFORTS/RELIEF MEASURES
		WARNING SIGNS
		FETAL ACTIVITY MONITORING
		LABOR SIGNS: WHEN AND HOW TO CALL
		TRAVEL RESTRICTIONS
		LABOR & DELIVERY ROUTINE
		ELECTRONIC FETAL MONITORING
		ANESTHESIA/ANALGESIA
		EPISIOTOMY/PERINEAL INTEGRITY
		LABOR & DELIVERY COMPLICATIONS/OPERATIVE DELIVERY
		BREAST CARE
		CAR SEAT
		DISCUSS POST-TERM MANAGEMENT
		EARLY DISCHARGE/HELP AT HOME

DATE	MEDICATIONS	POST PARTUM CONTRACEPTIVE PLANS
	RHOGAM	☐ ORAL CONTRACEPTION ☐ LONG ACTING CONTRACEPTION
		☐ STERILIZATION - DATE TUBAL FORM SIGNED _____
		☐ BARRIER ☐ OTHER
DRUG ALLERGIES/REACTIONS ☐ NKA		
PATIENT NAME		
		(Continued on page 290)

(Continued on page 290)

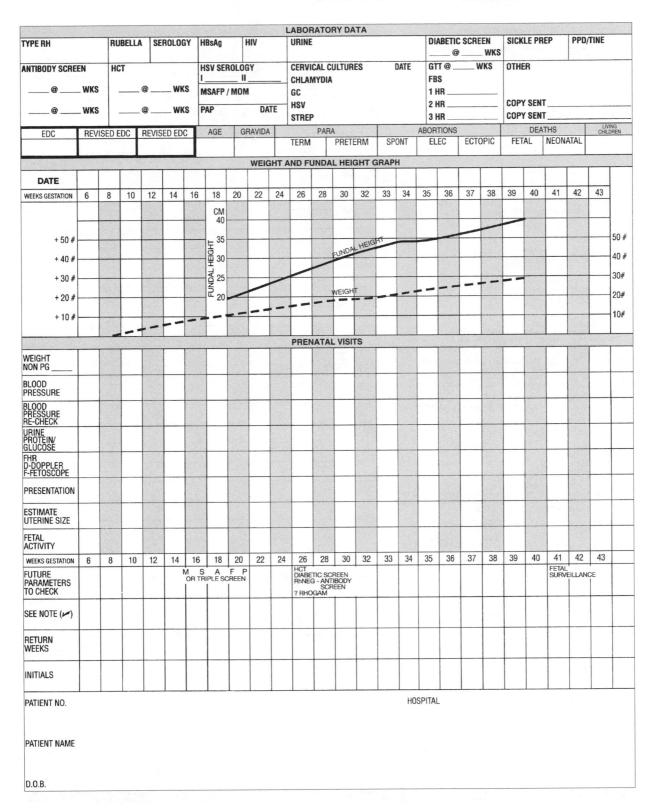

RISK FACTOR GUIDELINES	PROGRESS NOTES *(Continued from page 288)*

PATIENT PROFILE
AGE > 34 OR PREGNANCY WITHIN 2 YEARS OF MENARCHE
OCCUPATION AND AVOCATION
DRUG ABUSE OR ADDICTION
   ALCOHOL
   SMOKING
   COCAINE
   MARIJUANA
   NARCOTICS
   SEDATIVES/HYPNOTICS
   SALICYLATES AND OTHER PGSI'S
   OTHER
LOW SOCIO-ECONOMIC STATUS
   WELFARE
   EDUCATION < 9TH GRADE
   CROWDED LIVING CONDITIONS
   OTHER
BODY HABITUS
   SMALL STATURE (< 5 FEET TALL)
   OBESE (> 50# OVER IDEAL WEIGHT FOR HEIGHT)
   UNDERWEIGHT (> 20# UNDER IDEAL WEIGHT FOR HEIGHT)
   MATERNAL BIRTHWEIGHT (LOW BIRTHWEIGHT OR LARGE FOR DATES)
PARTNER
   MEDICAL OR SURGICAL DISORDERS
   DRUG, SMOKING OR ALCOHOL ABUSE
   OCCUPATION, AVOCATION, HOBBIES
   STD'S (HERPES, URETHRITIS)
   HIV RISK FACTORS

GYNECOLOGICAL HISTORY
UTERINE AND CERVICAL ABNORMALITIES
   PAST UTERINE SURGERY (NON-CESAREAN)
   UTERINE ANOMALIES (CONGENITAL ANOMALIES, DES STIGMATA, MYOMATA)
   CERVICAL LACERATIONS OR CONIZATIONS
MENSTRUAL HISTORY AND GESTATIONAL DATING
   IRREGULAR MENSES OR OLIGOAMENORRHEA
   ORAL CONTRACEPTIVE USE PRIOR TO CONCEPTION

MEDICAL HISTORY
   ANEMIA (HGB < 9.5 OR HCT < 30)
   HEART DISEASE (SYMPTOMATIC OR ASYMPTOMATIC)
   THROMBOEMBOLISM (DURING PREVIOUS PREGNANCY OR PRIOR TO
      CURRENT PREGNANCY)
   ANTICOAGULANT USE
   CHRONIC HYPERTENSION (BP > 140/90 AT FIRST PRENATAL VISIT)
   ASTHMA OR OTHER CHRONIC LUNG DISEASE
   SEIZURE DISORDER (WITH OR WITHOUT ANTICONVULSANT USE)
   DIABETES MELLITUS (GESTATIONAL OR PREGESTATIONAL)
   HEPATITIS
   HIV RISK FACTORS
   CHRONIC RENAL DISEASE (BUN > 20, CREATININE > 1.2 AT FIRST PRENATAL
      VISIT)
   PYELONEPHRITIS

OBSTETRICAL FACTORS
PARITY
   PRIMIGRAVIDA
   GRAND MULTIPARA (> 4)
PAST PREGNANCIES
   HABITUAL ABORTION ($\geq$ 3)
   PREMATURE BIRTH (< 37 WEEKS)
   PREMATURE RUPTURE OF MEMBRANES
   LOW BIRTH WEIGHT INFANT (BIRTHWEIGHT < 10TH PERCENTILE FOR DATES)
   LARGE FOR DATES INFANT (BIRTHWEIGHT > 90TH PERCENTILE FOR DATES)
   FETAL OR NEONATAL DEATH
   CONGENITAL ANOMALIES
   SURVIVING NEUROLOGICALLY IMPAIRED INFANT
   CERVICAL INCOMPETENCY
   MIDFORCEP OR DIFFICULT DELIVERY (E.G. SHOULDER DYSTOCIA)
   ABNORMAL LABOR (ARREST OR PROTRACTION DISORDER OF FIRST OR
      SECOND STAGE)
   ANTEPARTUM HEMORRHAGE (PLACENTAL ABRUPTION, PLACENTA PREVIA)
   BLEEDING PRIOR TO 20 WEEKS
   RH ISOIMMUNIZATION
   PREGNANCY INDUCED HYPERTENSION
   CESAREAN DELIVERY (LOW TRANSVERSE, LOW VERTICAL, CLASSICAL,
      UNKNOWN)
   INTERVAL FROM LAST DELIVERY < 12 MONTHS
   ANESTHESIA INTOLERANCE OR REACTIONS

PRESENT PREGNANCY
   EMOTIONAL STRESS
   POOR COMPLIANCE
   LATE REGISTRATION FOR CARE
   UNCERTAIN DATES
   FAILURE TO GAIN WEIGHT (< 1/2 # PER WEEK AFTER 12 WEEKS)
   EXCESSIVE WEIGHT GAIN (> 2 # PER WEEK AFTER 12 WEEKS)
   BLEEDING PRIOR TO 20 WEEKS
   LACK OF PREGNANCY NAUSEA AND VOMITING (MORNING SICKNESS)
   PLACENTAL ABRUPTION
   PLACENTA PREVIA
   OTHER VAGINAL BLEEDING
   PREMATURE RUPTURE OF MEMBRANES
   POLYHYDRAMNIOS OR OLIGOHYDRAMNIOS
   THREATENED PREMATURE LABOR

PATIENT NAME

RM 612 REV 5/97

UNIT 4

Integration of the Health Assessment

CHAPTER *28*

The Complete Health Assessment: Putting It All Together

PURPOSE

This chapter helps you to learn the methods of integrating the regional examinations so that you will be able to conduct a complete physical examination on a well young adult.

READING ASSIGNMENT

Jarvis, *Physical Examination and Health Assessment*, 4th ed., Chapter 28, pp. 835-856.

AUDIO-VISUAL ASSIGNMENT

Jarvis, *Saunders Video Series: Physical Examination and Health Assessment: Head-to-Toe Examination of the Adult*

CLINICAL OBJECTIVES

1. Demonstrate skills of inspection, percussion, palpation, and auscultation.

2. Demonstrate correct use of instruments, including assembly, manipulation of component parts, and positioning with patient.

3. Use appropriate terminology and correctly pronounce medical terminology with clinical instructor and with patient.

4. Choreograph the complete examination in a systematic manner, including integration of certain regional assessments throughout the examination (e.g., skin, musculoskeletal).

5. Coordinate procedures to limit position changes for examiner and patient.

6. Describe accurately the findings of the examination, including normal and abnormal findings.

7. Demonstrate appropriate infection control measures.

8. Recognize and maintain the privacy and dignity of the patient.

    a. Adequately explain what is being done while limiting small talk.
    b. Consider patient's anxiety and fears.
    c. Consider your own facial expression and comments.
    d. Demonstrate confidence, empathy, and gentle manner.
    e. Acknowledge and apologize for any discomfort caused.
    f. Provide for privacy and warmth at all times.
    g. Determine comfort level, pausing if patient becomes tired.
    h. Wash hands and don gloves appropriately.
    i. Allow adequate time for each step.
    j. Briefly summarize findings to patient, and thank patient for his or her time.

INSTRUCTIONS

The key to success in this venture is practice; you should conduct at least three complete physical examination practices in your preparation for this final examination proficiency. You are responsible for obtaining a peer "patient" for the examination. You should prepare your own note card "outline" for the examination. You may refer to this minimally during the examination, but over-dependence on your notes will constitute failure. You will have 45 minutes in which to conduct the examination (not including setup or genitalia examination). If you practice three times, you will have no difficulty completing the examination in the alloted time.

Prepare the examination setting. Arrange for proper lighting. If you are using a hospital bed instead of an examination table, make sure to adjust the bed height during the exam to allow for your own visualization of the patient, and for the patient's ease in getting into and out of the bed. Arrange adequate patient gown, bath blankets, and drapes.

Gather your equipment. The following items are needed for a complete physical examination, including female genitalia. Check with your clinical instructor for any items that you may omit for your own examination proficiency.

Platform scale with height attachment
Skinfold calipers
Sphygmomanometer with appropriate size cuff
Stethoscope with bell and diaphragm endpieces
Thermometer
Flashlight or penlight
Otoscope/ophthalmoscope
Tuning fork
Nasal speculum
Tongue depressor
Pocket vision screener
Skin-marking pen
Flexible tape measure and ruler marked in centimeters
Reflex hammer
Sharp object (split tongue blade)
Cotton balls
Bivalve vaginal speculum
Disposable gloves
Materials for cytologic study
Lubricant
Fecal occult blood test materials

Record your findings using the write-up sheets that follow. Your clinical instructor may ask you to record your findings ahead of time, following one of your practice sessions. Then you can give your write-up to the instructor to follow along as you perform the final examination proficiency.

Good luck!

Notes

COMPLETE PHYSICAL EXAMINATION

Date _____

Patient _____ **Age** _____ **Sex** _____ **Occupation** _____

Examiner _____

General Survey of Patient

1. Appears stated age
2. Level of consciousness _____
3. Skin color _____
4. Nutritional status _____
5. Posture and position _____
6. Obvious physical deformities _____
7. Mobility: gait, use of assistive devices, ROM of joints, no involuntary movement _____
8. Facial expression _____
9. Mood and affect _____
10. Speech: articulation, pattern, content appropriate, native language _____
11. Hearing _____
12. Personal hygiene _____

Measurement and Vital Signs

1. Weight _____
2. Height _____
3. Skinfold thickness, if indicated _____
4. Vision using Snellen eye chart _____
    OD _____ OS _____ Correction? _____
5. Radial pulse, rate, and rhythm _____
6. Respirations, rate, depth _____
7. Blood pressure
    Right arm _____(sitting or lying?)
    Left arm _____(sitting or lying?)
8. Temperature (if indicated) _____
9. Pain assessment _____

STAND IN FRONT OF PATIENT, PATIENT IS SITTING

Skin

1. Hands and nails _____
2. (For rest of exam, examine skin with corresponding region)
    Color and pigmentation _____
    Temperature _____
    Moisture _____
    Texture _____
    Turgor _____
    Any lesions _____

Head and Face

1. Scalp, hair, cranium _____
2. Face (cranial nerve VII) _____

Jarvis, Carolyn: PHYSICAL EXAMINATION AND HEALTH ASSESSMENT, Fourth Edition,
Student Laboratory Manual. Copyright © 2004, 2000, 1996, Elsevier Inc. All rights reserved.

3. Temporal artery, temporomandibular joint _____

4. Maxillary sinuses, frontal sinuses _____

Eyes

1. Visual fields (cranial nerve II) _____

2. Extraocular muscles, corneal light reflex
   Cardinal positions of gaze (cranial nerves III, IV, VI) _____

3. External structures _____

4. Conjunctivae _____
   Sclerae _____
   Corneas _____
   Irides _____

5. Pupils _____

6. Ophthalmoscope, red reflex _____
   Disc _____
   Vessels _____
   Retinal background _____

Ears

1. External ear _____

2. Any tenderness _____

3. Otoscope, ear canal _____
   Tympanic membrane _____

4. Test hearing (cranial nerve VIII), voice test _____
   Weber test _____
   Rinne test _____

Nose

1. External nose _____

2. Patency of nostrils _____

3. Speculum, nasal mucosa _____
   Septum _____
   Turbinates _____

Mouth and Throat

1. Lips and buccal mucosa _____
   Teeth and gums _____
   Tongue _____
   Hard/soft palate _____

2. Tonsils _____

3. Uvula (cranial nerves IX, X) _____

4. Tongue (cranial nerve XII) _____

Neck

1. Symmetry, lumps, pulsations _____
2. Cervical lymph nodes _____
3. Carotid pulse (bruits if indicated) _____
4. Trachea_____
5. ROM and muscle strength (cranial nerve XI)_____

MOVE TO BACK OF PATIENT, PATIENT SITTING

6. Thyroid gland _____

Chest and Lungs, Posterior and Lateral

1. Thoracic cage configuration _____
   Skin characteristics _____
   Symmetry _____
2. Symmetric expansion _____
   Tactile fremitus _____
   Lumps or tenderness _____
3. Spinous processes _____
4. Percussion over lung fields _____
   Diaphragmatic excursion _____
5. CVA tenderness _____
6. Breath sounds _____
7. Adventitious sounds _____

MOVE TO FRONT OF PATIENT

Chest and Lungs, Anterior

1. Respirations and skin characteristics _____
2. Tactile fremitus, lumps, tenderness _____
3. Percuss lung fields _____
4. Breath sounds _____

Upper Extremities

1. ROM and muscle strength _____
2. Epitrochlear nodes _____

Breasts

1. Symmetry, mobility, dimpling _____
2. Supraclavicular and infraclavicular areas _____

PATIENT SUPINE, STAND AT PATIENT'S RIGHT

3. Breast palpation _____
4. Nipple _____
5. Axillae and regional nodes _____
6. Teach breast self-examination _____

Neck Vessels

1. Jugular venous pulse _____
2. Jugular venous pressure, if indicated _____

Heart
1. Precordium: pulsations and heave _____
2. Apical impulse _____
3. Precordium, thrills _____
4. Apical rate and rhythm _____
5. Heart sounds _____

Abdomen
1. Contour, symmetry _____
   Skin characteristics _____
   Umbilicus and pulsations _____
2. Bowel sounds _____
3. Vascular sounds _____
4. Percussion _____
5. Liver span in right MCL _____
6. Spleen _____
7. Light and deep palpation _____
8. Palpation of liver, spleen, kidneys, aorta _____
9. Abdominal reflexes, if indicated _____

Inguinal Area
1. Femoral pulse _____
2. Inguinal nodes _____

Lower Extremities
1. Symmetry _____
   Skin characteristics, hair distribution _____
2. Pulses, popliteal _____
   Posterior tibial _____
   Dorsalis pedis _____
3. Temperature, pretibial edema _____
4. Toes _____

PATIENT SITS UP

5. ROM and muscle strength, hips _____
   Knees _____
   Ankles and feet _____

Neurologic
1. Sensation, face _____
   Arms and hands _____
   Legs and feet _____
2. Position sense _____
3. Stereognosis _____
4. Cerebellar function, finger-to-nose _____
5. Cerebellar function, heel-to-shin _____
6. Deep tendon reflexes
   Biceps _____ Triceps _____

Brachioradialis _____ Patellar _____
Achilles _____
7. Babinski reflex _____

PATIENT STANDS UP

Musculoskeletal
1. Walk across room _____
   Walk, heel to toe _____
2. Walk on tiptoes, then walk on heels _____
3. Romberg sign _____
4. Shallow knee bend _____
5. Touch toes _____
6. ROM of spine _____

Male Genitalia
1. Penis and scrotum _____
2. Testes and spermatic cord _____
3. Inguinal hernia _____
4. Teach testicular self-examination _____

Male Rectum
1. Perianal area _____
2. Rectal walls and prostate gland _____
3. Stool for occult blood _____

FEMALE PATIENT IN LITHOTOMY POSITION

Female Genitalia and Rectum
1. Perineal and perianal areas _____
2. Vaginal speculum: cervix and vaginal walls _____
3. Procure specimens _____
4. Bimanual: cervix, uterus, and adnexa _____
   _____
5. Rectovaginal _____
6. Stool for occult blood _____

HELP PATIENT SIT UP

THANK PATIENT FOR TIME, DEPART FROM PATIENT

Answers to Review Questions

CHAPTER 1

Critical Thinking in Health Assessment

1. a
2. d
3. c
4. b
5. c
6. a

CHAPTER 2

Developmental Tasks and Health Promotion Across the Life Cycle

1. c
2. b
3. a
4. d
5. c
6. d
7. d
8. c
9. a
10. c
11. b
12. b

CHAPTER 3

Transcultural Considerations in Assessment

1. b
2. c
3. a
4. c
5. b
6. a

CHAPTER 4

The Interview

1. a
2. a
3. b
4. c
5. d
6. b
7. a
8. d
9. b
10. d
11. b
12. c
13. a

CHAPTER 5

Domestic Violence Assessment

1. d
2. a
3. b
4. b
5. a
6. e

CHAPTER 6

The Complete Health History

1. d
2. a
3. c
4. b
5. c
6. c
7. a
8. d
9. b
10. d

CHAPTER 7

Mental Status Assessment

1. d
2. a

3. d

4. c

5. b

6. c

7. b

8. c

9. a

10. c

11. i

12. d

13. b

14. g

15. f

16. a

17. e

18. h

19. Patient is dressed and groomed appropriately for season and setting. Posture is erect, with no involuntary body movements. Oriented to time, person, and place. Recent and remote memory intact. Affect and verbal responses appropriate. Perceptions and thought processes logical and coherent.

CHAPTER 8

Nutritional Assessment

1. c

2. d

3. c

4. c

5. c

6. b

7. b

8. a

9. b

10. c

11. c

12. d

CHAPTER 9

Assessment Techniques and the Clinical Setting

1. d

2. c

3. b

4. a

5. c

6. d

7. c

8. c

CHAPTER 10

General Survey, Measurement, Vital Signs

1. d

2. c

3. b

4. a

5. c

6. a

7. b

8. b

9. d

10. a

11. d

12. c

CHAPTER 11

Pain Assessment: the Fifth Vital Sign

1. c

2. b

3. c

4. d

5. d

6. b

7. c

8. b

9. d

10. c

11. d

12. b

CHAPTER 12

Skin, Hair, and Nails

1. b

2. d

3. a

4. d

5. b

6. d

7. c

8. c

9. a

10. c

11. d

12. c

13. c

14. c

15. a

16. b

17. a

18. c

19. b

20. c

21. a

22. a

23. b

24. c

25. a
26. b
27. d
28. b
29. a
30. g
31. c
32. f
33. d
34. e

CHAPTER 13

Head and Neck, Including Regional Lymphatics

1. d
2. c
3. b
4. a
5. d
6. d
7. c
8. d
9. a
10. a
11. a
12. c
13. c
14. e
15. f
16. h
17. g
18. i
19. j
20. b
21. d
22. a

CHAPTER 14

Eyes

1. b
2. c
3. a
4. b
5. d
6. c
7. a
8. c
9. a
10. c
11. b
12. c
13. b
14. a
15. b
16. Instruct the patient to hold the head steady and follow the examiner's finger. The examiner holds the finger 12 inches from the individual and moves it clockwise to the positions of 2, 3, 4, 8, 9, and 10 o'clock and back to the center each time. A normal response is parallel tracking of the object with both eyes.

CHAPTER 15

Ears

1. c
2. a
3. d
4. b
5. a
6. c

7. c
8. d
9. b
10. d
11. b
12. a
13. b
14. b
15. a
16. d

CHAPTER 16

Nose, Mouth, and Throat

1. c
2. d
3. a
4. a
5. b
6. a
7. b
8. d
9. c
10. a
11. d
12. a

CHAPTER 17

Breasts and Regional Lymphatics

1. d
2. b
3. a
4. c
5. a
6. c
7. c
8. c

9. b
10. d
11. c
12. b
13. d
14. a
15. b

CHAPTER 18

Thorax and Lungs

1. a
2. b
3. b
4. a
5. c
6. b
7. b
8. d
9. c
10. d
11. b
12. c
13. a
14. e
15. a
16. c
17. d
18. b
19. e
20. a
21. d
22. f
23. c
24. b

CHAPTER 19

Heart and Neck Vessels

1. c
2. b
3. c
4. b
5. d
6. d
7. b
8. b
9. a
10. a
11. a
12. b
13. c
14. c
15. e
16. c
17. f
18. a
19. b
20. d
21. Liver to right atrium via inferior vena cava, through tricuspid valve to right ventricle, through the pulmonic valve to the pulmonary artery, picks up oxygen in the lungs, returns to left atrium, to left ventricle via mitral valve, through aortic valve to aorta and out to the body.
22. The major risk factors for heart disease and stroke are hypertension, smoking, high cholesterol levels, obesity, and diabetes. Physical inactivity, family history of heart disease, and age are other risk factors.

CHAPTER 20

Peripheral Vascular System and Lymphatic System

1. a
2. c
3. c
4. b
5. c
6. d
7. a
8. d
9. b
10. d
11. a
12. c
13. a
14. c

CHAPTER 21

Abdomen

1. c
2. c
3. a
4. d
5. c
6. a
7. d
8. d
9. d
10. a

11. d

12. a

13. c

14. b

CHAPTER 22

Musculoskeletal System

1. d

2. b

3. d

4. c

5. d

6. a

7. a

8. c

9. b

10. The musculoskeletal system provides support to the body, enabling it to stand erect and to move. The system protects inner organs, produces red blood cells, and provides for the storage of minerals.

11. b

12. e

13. g

14. i

15. d

16. a

17. j

18. m

19. k

20. n

21. l

22. h

23. f

24. c

CHAPTER 23

Neurologic System

1. a

2. d

3. c

4. c

5. b

6. c

7. b

8. a

9. b

10. d

11. b

12. c

13. f

14. b

15. g

16. k

17. h

18. c

19. l

20. d

21. i

22. e

23. j

24. a

CHAPTER 24

Male Genitalia

1. c

2. c

3. d

4. c

5. c

6. d

7. b

8. a

9. d

10. a

11. a

12. b

13. e

14. Voids clear, amber urine 5 to 6 times a day. No nocturia, dysuria, or hesitancy. No pain or discharge from penis. Sexually active with multiple partners. Uses prophylaxis that is satisfactory for both partners. No history of sexually transmitted disease. No lesions, inflammation, or discharge from penis noted on examination. Testes descended without masses. No inguinal hernia.

CHAPTER 25

Anus, Rectum, and Prostate

1. a

2. b

3. c

4. a

5. d

6. c

7. b

8. c

9. a

10. No recent change in bowel habits. One BM daily, soft, dark brown in color. No pain or bleeding. No medications. Diet includes 4 servings of fruits and vegetables daily. No hemorrhoids or rectal lesions noted. Sphincter tone good. No masses or tenderness on palpation. No masses, tenderness, or enlargement of prostate. Stool is Hematest negative.

CHAPTER 26

Female Genitalia

1. d
2. a
3. d
4. c
5. c
6. d
7. d
8. b
9. c
10. b
11. b
12. a
13. a
14. Menarche at age 14, cycle 28 to 32 days of 4–5 days duration. Flow moderate with no dysmenorrhea. Gravida 0/Para 0/Ab 0. Has annual Gyn exam. No urinary problems, no vaginal discharge. Uses barrier method of birth control. Method satisfactory to self and partner.

CHAPTER 27

The Pregnant Female

1. c
2. a
3. c
4. a
5. c
6. c
7. b
8. e
9. f
10. f
11. d
12. b
13. c
14. d
15. f
16. Possible answers include:

   1) Fundal height small for dates. Possible causes: innacurate dates, premature labor, intrauterine growth restriction, fetal position

   2) Fundal height larger for dates. Possible causes: inaccurate dates, hydatidiform mole, multiple fetuses, polyhydramnios, fetal macrosomia

   3) Vaginal bleeding. Possible causes: blighted ovum, friable cervix, ectopic pregnancy, perigestational hemorrhage, cervical lesions, threatened miscarriage, placenta previa, abruptio placentae, uterine rupture

APPENDIX

Summary of Infant Growth and Development

AGE (MOS)	PHYSICAL COMPETENCY	INTELLECTUAL COMPETENCY	EMOTIONAL-SOCIAL COMPETENCY
1 to 2	Holds head in alignment when prone; Moro reflex to loud sound; follows objects; smiles	Reflex activity; vowel sounds produced	Gratification through sucking and basic needs being promptly met; smiles at people
2 to 4	Turns back to side; raises head and chest 45–90 degrees off bed and supports weight on arms; reaches for objects; follows object through midline; drools; begins to localize sounds; prefers configuration of face	Reproduces behavior initially achieved by random activity; imitates behavior previously done. Visually studies objects; locates sounds; makes cooing sounds; does not look for objects removed from presence	Social responsiveness; awareness of those who are not primary care giver; smiles in response to familiar face
4 to 6	Birth weight doubled; teeth eruption may begin; sits with stable head and back control; rolls from abdomen to back; picks up object with palmar grasp	Some intentional actions; some sense of object permanence, looks on same path for vanished object; recognizes partially hidden objects; more systematic in imitative behavior; babbles	Prefers primary care giver; sucking needs decrease; laughs in pleasure
6 to 8	Turns back to stomach; sits alone; crawls; transfers objects hand to hand; turns to sound behind	Continued development as in 4 to 6 months	Differentiated response to nonprimary care takers; evidence of "stranger" or "separation" anxiety
8 to 10	Creeps; pulls to stand; pincer grasp	Actions more goal directed; able to solve simple problems by using previously mastered responses. Actively searches for an object that disappears	Attachment process complete
10 to 12	Birth weight tripled; cruises; stands by self; may use spoon	Begins to imitate behavior done before by others but not by self. Understands words being said; may say 1 to 4 words. Intentionality is present	Begins to explore and separate briefly from parent

Appendix continues on following page

(Modified from Betz C, Hunsberger M, Wright S: Family-Centered Nursing Care of Children, 2nd ed. Philadelphia, WB Saunders, 1994, pp 148-149. Used with permission.)

	NUTRITION	PLAY	SAFETY
1 to 2	Breastfed or fortified formula	Variety of positions. Care taker should hold and talk to infant, large, brightly colored objects	Car carrier; proper use of infant seat
2 to 4	As for 1 to 2 months	Talk to and hold. Musical toys; rattle, mobile. Variety of objects of different color, size, and texture; mirror, crib toys, variety of settings	Do not leave unattended on couch, bed, etc. Remove any small objects that infant could choke on
4 to 6	Introduction of solids; initial store of iron depletion	Talk and hold. Provide open space to move and objects to grasp	Keep environment free of safety hazards; check toys for sharp edges and small pieces that might break
6 to 8	As for 4 to 6 months	Provide place to explore. Stack toys, blocks; nursery rhymes	Check infant's expanding environment for hazards
8 to 10	As for 4 to 6 months	Games: hide and seek; peek-a-boo, pat-a-cake, looking at pictures in a book Do not leave alone in bathtub Keep poisons out of reach and locked up Continue use of safety seat in car	Keep: electrical outlets plugged, cords out of reach, stairs blocked, coffee and end tables cleared of hazards
10 to 12	More solids than liquids; increasing use of cup; begin to wean	Increase space; read to infant. Name and point to body parts. Water; sand play; ball	As for 8 to 10 months

APPENDIX

Summary of Toddler Growth, Development, and Health Maintenance

AGE (MOS)	PHYSICAL COMPETENCY	INTELLECTUAL COMPETENCY	EMOTIONAL-SOCIAL COMPETENCY
General: 1 to 3 yrs	Gains 5 kg (11 lb) Grows 20.3 cm (8 in) 12 teeth erupt Nutritional requirements: Energy 100 Kcal/kg/day Fluid 115–125 ml/kg/day Protein 1.8 gm/kg/day See Chapter 6 for vitamins and minerals.	Learns by exploring and experimenting Learns by imitating. Progresses from a vocabulary of three to four words at 12 months to about 900 words at 36 months.	Central crisis: to gain a sense of autonomy versus doubt and shame. Demonstrates independent behaviors. Exhibits attachment behavior strongly and regularly until third birthday. Fears persist of strange people, objects, and places and of aloneness and being abandoned. Egocentric in play (parallel play). Imitation of parents in household tasks and activities of daily living.
15 mos	Legs appear bowed. Walks alone, climbs, slides downstairs backward. Stacks two blocks. Scribbles spontaneously. Grasps spoon but rotates it, holds cup with both hands. Takes off socks and shoes.	Trial and error method of learning. Experiments to see what will happen. Says at least three words. Uses expressive jargon.	Shows independence by trying to feed self and helps in undressing.
18 mos	Runs but still falls. Walks upstairs with help. Slides downstairs backwards. Stacks three to four blocks. Clumsily throws a ball. Unzips a large zipper. Takes off simple garments.	Begins to maintain a mental image of an absent object. Concept of object permanence fully develops. Has vocabulary of 10 or more words. Holophrastic speech (one word used to communicate whole ideas)	Fears the water. Temper tantrums may begin. Negativism and dawdling predominate. Bedtime rituals begin. Awareness of gender identity begins. Helps with undressing.

Appendix continues on following page

(From Betz C, Hunsberger M, Wright S: Family-Centered Nursing Care of Children, 2nd ed. Philadelphia, WB Saunders, 1994, pp 190–191. Used with permission.)

AGE	PHYSICAL COMPETENCY	INTELLECTUAL COMPETENCY	EMOTIONAL-SOCIAL COMPETENCY
24 mos	Runs quickly and with fewer falls. Pulls toys and walks sideways. Walks downstairs hanging on a rail (does not alternate feet). Stacks six blocks. Turns pages of a book. Imitates vertical and circular strokes. Uses spoon with little spilling. Can feed self. Puts on simple garments. Can turn door knobs.	Enters into preconceptual phase of preoperational period: Symbolic thinking and symbolic play. Egocentric thinking, imagination, and pretending are common. Has vocabulary of about 300 words. Uses two-word sentences (telegraphic speech). Engages in monologue.	Fears the dark and animals. Temper tantrums may continue. Negativism and dawdling continue. Bedtime rituals continue. Sleep resisted overtly. Usually shows readiness to begin bowel and bladder control. Explores genitalia. Brushes teeth with help. Helps with dressing and undressing.
36 mos	Has set of deciduous teeth at about 30 months. Walks downstairs alternating feet. Rides tricycle. Walks with balance and runs well. Stacks eight to ten blocks. Can pour from a pitcher. Feeds self completely. Dresses self almost completely (does not know front from back). Cannot tie shoes.	Preconceptual phase of preoperational period as for 24 months. Uses around 900 words. Constructs complete sentences and uses all parts of speech.	Temper tantrums subside. Negativism and dawdling subside. Bedtime rituals subside. Self-care in feeding, elimination and dressing enhances self-esteem.

	NUTRITION	PLAY	SAFETY
General: 1 to 3 yrs	Milk 16–24 oz. Appetite decreases. Wants to feed self. Has food jags. Never force food; give nutritious snacks. Give iron and vitamin supplementation only if poor intake.	Books at all stages. Needs physical and quiet activities, does not need expensive toys.	Never leave alone in tub. Keep poisons, including detergents and cleaning products, out of reach. Use car seat. Have ipecac in house.
15 mos	Vulnerable to iron deficiency anemia. Give table foods except for tough meat and hard vegetables. Wants to feed self.	Stuffed animals, dolls, music toys. Peek-a-boo, hide and seek. Water and sand play. Stacking toys. Roll ball on floor. Push toys on floor. Read to toddler.	Keep small items off floor (pins, buttons, clips). Child may choke on hard food. Cords and tablecloths are a danger. Keep electrical outlets plugged and poisons locked away. Risk of kitchen accidents with toddler under foot.
18 mos	Negativism may interfere with eating. Encourage self-feeding. Is easily distracted while eating. May play with food. High activity level interferes with eating.	Rocking horse. Nesting toys. Shapesorting cube. Pencil or crayon. Pull toys. Four-wheeled toy ride. Throw ball. Running and chasing games. Rough-housing. Puzzles. Blocks. Hammer and peg board.	Falls: from riding toy in bathtub from running too fast Climbs up to get dangerous objects. Keep dangerous things out of waste-basket.
24 mos	Requests certain foods; therefore snacks should be controlled. Imitates eating habits of others. May still play with food and especially with utensils and dish (pouring, stacking).	Clay and Play-Doh. Finger paint. Brush paint. Record player with record and story book and songs to sing along. Toys to take apart. Toy tea sets. Puppets. Puzzles.	May fall from outdoor large play equipment. Can reach farther than expected (knives, razors, and matches must be kept out of reach).
36 mos	Sits in booster seat rather than high chair. Verbal about likes and dislikes.	Likes playing with other children, building toys, drawing and painting, doing puzzles. Imitation household objects for doll play. Nurse and doctor kits. Carpenter kits.	Protect from: turning on hot water falling from tricycle striking matches.

APPENDIX

Growth, Development, and Health Promotion for Preschoolers

AGE (YRS)	PHYSICAL COMPETENCY	INTELLECTUAL COMPETENCY	EMOTIONAL-SOCIAL COMPETENCY
General: 3 to 5	Gains 4.5 kg (10 lb) Grows 15 cm (6 in) 20 teeth present Nutritional requirements: Energy: 1250 to 1600 cal/day (or 90 to 100 Kcal/kg/day) Fluid: 100 to 125 ml/kg/day Protein: 30 g/day (or 3 g/kg/day) Iron: 10 mg/day	Becomes increasingly aware of self and others Vocabulary increases from 900 to 2100 words Piaget's preoperational/intuitive period	Freud's phallic stage Oedipus complex—boy Electra complex—girl Erikson's stage of Initiative vs. Guilt
3	Runs, stops suddenly Walks backward Climbs steps Jumps Pedals tricycle Undresses self Unbuttons front buttons Feeds self well	Knows own sex Sense of humor Desires to please Language—900 words Follows simple direction Uses plurals Names figure in picture Uses adjectives/adverbs	Shifts between reality and imagination Bedtime rituals Negativism decreases Animism and realism: anything that moves is alive
4	Runs well, skips clumsily Hops on one foot Heel-toe walk Up and down steps without holding rail Jumps well Dresses and undresses Buttons well, needs help with zippers, bows Brushes teeth Bathes self Draws with some form and meaning	More aware of others Uses alibis to excuse behavior Bossy Language—1500 words Talks in sentences Knows nursery rhymes Counts to 5 Highly imaginative Name calling	Focuses on present Egocentrism/unable to see the view point of others, unable to understand another's inability to see own viewpoint Does not comprehend anticipatory explanation Sexual curiosity Oedipus complex Electra complex

Appendix continues on following page

(From Betz C, Hunsberger M, Wright S: Family-Centered Nursing Care of Children, 2nd ed. Philadelphia, WB Saunders, 1994, pp 235-236. Used with permission.)

AGE (YRS)	PHYSICAL COMPETENCY	INTELLECTUAL COMPETENCY	EMOTIONAL-SOCIAL COMPETENCY
5	Runs skillfully Jumps 3–4 steps Jumps rope, hops, skips Begins dance Roller skates Dresses without assistance Ties shoelaces Hits nail on head with hammer Draws person—6 parts Prints first name	Aware of cultural differences Knows name and address More independent More sensible/less imaginative Copies triangle, draws rectangle Knows four or more colors Language—2100 words, meaningful sentences Understands kinship Counts to 10	Continues in egocentrism Fantasy and daydreams Resolution of Oedipus/Electra complex, girls identify with mother, boys with father Body image and body boundary especially important in illness Shows tension in nail-biting, nose-picking, whining, snuffling

	NUTRITION	PLAY	SAFETY
General: 3 to 5	Carbohydrate intake approximately 40 to 50 percent of calories Good food sources of essential vitamins and minerals Regular tooth brushing Parents are seen as examples; if parent won't eat it, child won't	Reading books is important at all ages Balance highly physical activities with quiet times Quiet rest period takes the place of nap time Provide sturdy play materials	Never leave alone in bath or swimming pool Keep poisons in locked cupboard; learn what household things are poisonous Use car seats and seatbelts Never leave child alone in car Remove doors from abandoned refrigerators
3	1250 cal/day Due to increased sex identity and imitation, copies parents at table and will eat what they eat Different colors and shapes of foods can increase interest	Participates in simple games Cooperates, takes turns Plays with group Uses scissors, paper Likes crayons, coloring books Enjoys being read to and "reading" Plays "dress-up" and "house" Likes fire engines	Teach safety habits early Let water out of bathtub; don't stand in tub Caution against climbing in unsafe areas, onto or under cars, unsafe buildings, drainage pipes Insist on seatbelts worn at all times in cars

	NUTRITION	PLAY	SAFETY
4	Good nutrition 1400 cal/day Nutritious between-meal snacks essential Emphasis on quality not quantity of food eaten Mealtime should be enjoyable, not for criticism As dexterity improves, neatness increases	Longer attention span with group activities "Dress-up" with more dramatic play Draws, pounds, paints Likes to make paper chains, sewing cards Scrapbooks Likes being read to, records, and rhythmic play "Helps" adults	Teach to stay out of streets, alleys Continually teach safety; child understands Teach how to handle scissors Teach what are poisons and why to avoid Never allow child to stand in moving car
5	Good nutrition 1600 cal/day Encourage regular tooth brushing Encourage quiet time before meals Can learn to cut own meat Frequent illnesses from increased exposure increase nutritional needs	Plays with trucks, cars, soldiers, dolls Likes simple games with letters or numbers Much gross motor activity: water, mud, snow, leaves, rocks Matching picture games	Teach child how to cross streets safely Teach child not to speak to strangers or get into cars of strangers Insist on seatbelts Teach child to swim

APPENDIX

Competency Development of the School-Aged Child

AGE (YRS)	PHYSICAL COMPETENCY	INTELLECTUAL COMPETENCY	EMOTIONAL-SOCIAL COMPETENCY
General: 6 to 12	Gains an average of 2.5 to 3.2 kg/year (5 1/2 to 7 lbs/year). Overall height gains of 5.5 cm (2 in) per year; growth occurs in spurts and is mainly in trunk and extremities. Loses deciduous teeth; most of permanent teeth erupt. Progressively more coordinated in both gross and fine motor skills. Caloric needs increase with growth spurts.	Masters concrete operations. Moves from egocentrism; learns he or she is not always right. Learns grammar and expression of emotions and thoughts. Vocabulary increases to 3000 words or more; handles complex sentences.	Central crisis: industry vs. inferiority; wants to do and make things. Progressive sex education needed. Wants to be like friends; competition important. Fears body mutilation, alterations in body image; earlier phobias may recur, nightmares; fears death. Nervous habits common.
6 to 7	Gross motor skill exceeds fine motor coordination. Balance and rhythm are good—runs, skips, jumps, climbs, gallops. Throws and catches ball. Dresses self with little or no help.	Vocabulary of 2500 words. Learning to read and print; beginning concrete concepts of numbers, general classification of items. Knows concepts of right and left; morning, afternoon, and evening; coinage. Intuitive thought process. Verbally aggressive, bossy, opinionated, argumentative. Likes simple games with basic rules.	Boisterous, outgoing, and a know-it-all, whiney; parents should sidestep power struggles, offer choices. Becomes quiet and reflective during seventh year; very sensitive. Can use telephone. Likes to make things: starts many, finishes few. Give some responsibility for household duties.
8 to 10	Myopia may appear. Secondary sex characteristics begin in girls. Hand-eye coordination and fine motor skills well established. Movements are graceful, coordinated. Cares for own physical needs completely. Constantly on move; plays and works hard; enforce balance in rest and activity.	Learning correct grammar and to express feelings in words. Likes books he or she can read alone; will read funny papers, scan newspaper. Enjoys making detailed drawings. Mastering classification, seriation, spatial and temporal, numerical concepts. Uses language as a tool; likes riddles, jokes, chants, word games. Rules guiding force in life now. Very interested in how things work, what and how weather, seasons, etc., are made.	Strong preference for same-sex peers; antagonizes opposite-sex peers. Self-assured and pragmatic at home; questions parental values and ideas. Has a strong sense of humor. Enjoys clubs, group projects, outings, large groups, camp. Modesty about own body increases over time; sex conscious. Works diligently to perfect skills he or she does best. Happy, cooperative, relaxed, and casual in relationships. Increasingly courteous and well-mannered with adults. Gang stage at a peak; secret codes and rituals prevail. Responds better to suggestion than dictatorial approach.

Appendix continues on following page

(From Betz C, Hunsberger M, Wright S; Family-Centered Nursing Care of Children, 2nd ed. Philadelphia, WB Saunders, 1994, pp 281-282. Used with permission.)

AGE (YRS)	PHYSICAL COMPETENCY	INTELLECTUAL COMPETENCY	EMOTIONAL-SOCIAL COMPETENCY
11 to 12	Vital signs approximate adult norms. Growth spurt for girls; inequalities between sexes are increasingly noticeable; boys have greater physical strength. Eruption of permanent teeth complete except for third molars. Secondary sex characteristics begin in boys. Menstruation may begin.	Able to think about social problems and prejudices; sees others' points of view. Enjoys reading mysteries, love stories. Begins playing with abstract ideas. Interested in whys of health measures and understands human reproduction. Very moralistic; religious commitment often made during this time.	Intense team loyalty; boys begin teasing girls and girls flirt with boys for attention; best friend period. Wants unreasonable independence. Rebellious about routine; wide mood swings; needs some time daily for privacy. Very critical of own work. Hero worship prevails. "Facts of life" chats with friends prevail; masturbation increases. Appears under constant tension.

	NUTRITION	PLAY	SAFETY
General: 6 to 12	Fluctuations in appetite due to uneven growth pattern and tendency to get involved in activities. Tendency to neglect breakfast owing to rush of getting to school. Though school lunch is provided in most schools, child does not always eat it.	Plays in groups, mostly of same sex; "gang" activities predominate. Books for all ages. Bicycles important. Sports equipment. Cards, board and table games. Most of play is active games requiring little or no equipment.	Enforce continued use of safety belts during car travel. Bicycle safety must be taught and enforced. Teach safety related to hobbies, handicrafts, mechanical equipment.
6 to 7	Preschool food dislikes persist. Tendency for deficiencies in iron, vitamin A, and riboflavin. 100 ml/kg of water per day. 3 gm/kg protein daily.	Still enjoys dolls, cars, and trucks. Plays well alone but enjoys small groups of both sexes; begins to prefer same sex peer during 7th year. Ready to learn how to ride a bicycle. Prefers imaginary, dramatic play with real costumes. Begins collecting for quantity, not quality. Enjoys active games such as hide-and-seek, tag, jumprope, roller skating, kickball. Ready for lessons in dancing, gymnastics, music. Restrict TV time to 1-2 hours/day.	Teach and reinforce traffic safety. Still needs adult supervision of play. Teach to avoid strangers, never take anything from strangers. Teach illness prevention and reinforce continued practice of other health habits. Restrict bicycle use to home ground; no traffic areas; teach bicycle safety. Teach the harmful use of drugs, alcohol, smoking. Set a good example.
8 to 10	Needs about 2100 calories/day; nutritious snacks. Tends to be too busy to bother to eat. Tendency for deficiencies in calcium, iron, and thiamine. Problem of obesity may begin now. Good table manners. Able to help with food preparation.	Likes hiking, sports. Enjoys cooking, woodworking, crafts. Enjoys cards and table games. Likes radio and records. Begins qualitative collecting now. Continue restriction on TV time.	Stress safety with firearms. Keep them out of reach and allow use only with adult supervision. Know who the child's friends are; parents should still have some control over friend selection. Teach water safety; swimming should be supervised by an adult.
11 to 12	Male needs 2500 calories per day; female needs 2250 (70 cal/kg/day). 75 ml/kg of water per day. 2 gm/kg protein daily.	Enjoys projects and working with hands. Likes to do errands and jobs to earn money. Very involved in sports, dancing, talking on phone. Enjoys all aspects of acting and drama.	Continue monitoring friends; stress bicycle safety on streets and in traffic.

APPENDIX

Characteristics of Adolescents

EARLY ADOLESCENCE (12 TO 14 YR)	MIDDLE ADOLESCENCE (15 TO 16 YR)	LATE ADOLESCENCE (17 TO 21 YR)
Becomes comfortable with own body; egocentric Difficulty solving problems; thinks in present; cannot use past experience to control behavior; sense of invulnerability—society's rules do not apply to him or her Struggle between dependent and independent behavior; begins forming peer alliance Parent-child conflict begins; teen argues but without logic	"Tries out" adultlike behavior Begins to solve problems, analyze, and abstract Established peer group alliance with associated risk-taking behavior Peak turmoil in child-family relations; able to debate issues and use some logic but not continuously	Aware of own strengths and limitations; establishes own value system Able to verbalize conceptually: deals with abstract moral concepts; makes decisions re future Peer group diminishes in importance; may develop first intimate relationship Turbulence subsides. May move away from home. More adultlike friendship with parents

(From Foster R, Hunsberger M, Anderson JJ: Family-Centered Nursing Care of Children. Philadelphia, WB Saunders, 1989, p. 359. Used with permission.)

APPENDIX

Functional Health Patterns Guide

The following table is a general guide for programs employing a functional health patterns approach to assessment.

Functional Health Patterns	Potential Correlating Chapters in the Text
Health Perception—Health Management	• Chapter 2, Developmental Tasks and Health Promotion Across the Life Cycle • Chapter 4, The Interview • Chapter 6, The Complete Health History
Nutritional—Metabolic	• Chapter 8, Nutritional Assessment • Chapter 10, General Survey, Measurement, Vital Signs • Chapter 12, Skin, Hair, and Nails • Chapter 16, Nose, Mouth, and Throat • Chapter 21, Abdomen
Elimination '	• Chapter 21, Abdomen • Chapter 24, Male Genitalia • Chapter 25, Anus, Rectum, and Prostate • Chapter 26, Female Genitalia
Activity—Exercise	• Chapter 18, Thorax and Lungs • Chapter 19, Heart and Neck Vessels • Chapter 20, Peripheral Vascular System and Lymphatic System • Chapter 22, Musculoskeletal System
Sleep—Rest	Chapter 6, The Complete Health History
Cognitive—Perception	• Chapter 7, Mental Status Assessment • Chapter 11, Pain Assessment: the Fifth Vital Sign • Chapter 13, Head and Neck, Including Regional Lymphatics • Chapter 14, Eyes • Chapter 15, Ears • Chapter 16, Nose, Mouth, and Throat • Chapter 23, Neurologic System

Self-Perception—Self-Concept	• Chapter 2, Developmental Tasks and Health Promotion Across the Life Cycle • Chapter 7, Mental Status Assessment
Role—Relationship	• Chapter 2, Developmental Tasks and Health Promotion Across the Life Cycle • Chapter 3, Transcultural Considerations in Assessment • Chapter 5, Domestic Violence Assessment
Sexuality—Reproductive	• Chapter 17, Breasts and Regional Lymphatics • Chapter 24, Male Genitalia • Chapter 26, Female Genitalia • Chapter 27, The Pregnant Female
Coping—Stress Tolerance	Chapter 2, Developmental Tasks and Health Promotion Across the Life Cycle
Value—Belief	• Chapter 2, Developmental Tasks and Health Promotion Across the Life Cycle • Chapter 3, Transcultural Considerations in Assessment